A TRADITION OF CHOICE

PLANNED PARENTHOOD AT 75

Planned Parenthood Federation of America, Inc., New York, New York 1991

A Tradition of Choice
Planned Parenthood® at 75

© Copyright 1991
Planned Parenthood Federation of America, Inc.

Printed in the United States of America

To order this publication (PPFA Item #1967), contact:
    Marketing Department
    Planned Parenthood Federation of America, Inc.
    810 Seventh Avenue
    New York, New York 10019

Library of Congress Catalog Card Number: 91-75358

ISBN 0-934586-71-3

PPFA Katharine Dexter McCormick Library
Classification 2.7

8/91-10

*T*his book is dedicated to continuing the struggle for reproductive freedom and women's rights to which noted attorney Harriet Fleischl Pilpel devoted nearly 60 years of her life and in which she was fully engaged at the time of her death in 1991.

FOREWORD BY KATHARINE HEPBURN

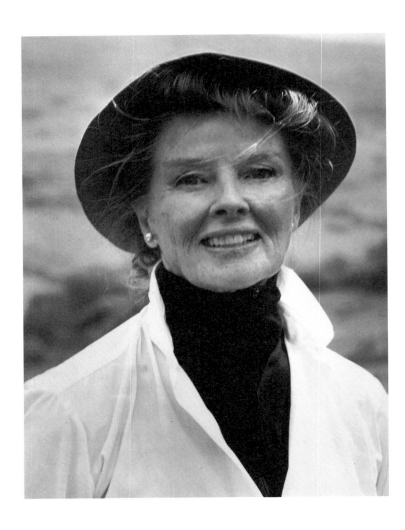

I can't think of anything more essential to women's self-determination, more crucial to personal fulfillment, or more basic to sexual equality than reproductive freedom. The struggle for reproductive freedom is a struggle I was *born* to. It is one of the most precious legacies I received from the two fascinating individuals who happened to be my parents. My mother and father were among the earliest and most passionate champions of the American family planning movement. My father, Dr. Thomas N. Hepburn, was a urologist. Appalled by the number of his patients who suffered the devastating effects of venereal disease, he helped to found the Connecticut Social Hygiene Association. ("Social hygiene" was the polite term, in those days, for efforts to curb sexually transmitted diseases — one of Planned Parenthood's important goals for 75 years now.)

My mother, Katharine Houghton Hepburn, came to the family planning movement through her work as an ardent suffragist. She knew that birth control was as essential to women's emancipation as the vote itself. As early as 1911, Mother launched a campaign for birth control in her Connecticut hometown. In 1923, she and some friends founded the Connecticut Birth Control League, which later became Planned Parenthood of Connecticut. And in 1928, she joined Margaret Sanger in building a new, controversial organization called the American Birth Control League. Today that organization is known as the Planned Parenthood Federation of America.

Mother's partnership with Margaret Sanger was among the most fulfilling elements of her life. I think one of her proudest moments must have been after a successful fund raiser, when Margaret Sanger commented about her, "Kate does it all, and perfectly."

So, as far back as I can remember, both Mother and Dad were constantly engrossed in improving sexual health and women's rights, especially for the poor and defenseless. With parents like these, it was inevitable that I would become an activist at an early age!

I remember childhood days at the Connecticut fairgrounds, where my mother's suffragettes always had a booth. I was in charge of the balloons — "Votes for Women" balloons, purple, white, and green. I used to take them into the fairgrounds and pursue some poor visitor until they finally accepted a balloon. In a rather insistent little voice, I'd say, "Votes for women! Here, take it! Votes for women!"... And they took it!

The significance of reproductive freedom came to me a little later in life. When I was first told about sex, I remember thinking, "I can't ever imagine wanting to do that with *anyone!*" Naturally, my feelings matured some as I grew! As a young woman, I had a beau who was considerably older than I. Daddy took him aside once and said, "I must give you some serious advice. My daughter is like a young bull about to charge...but if you lay hands on her, I'll shoot you." The man left town.

Quite obviously, I was very lucky to have my parents. They taught me that all women and men are endowed with dignity and responsibility. When a woman is faced with a sexual or reproductive decision, I cannot for the life of me see that anyone but that woman has the right to decide what she's going to do. That's what the birth control movement is all about.

The work begun by my parents and Margaret Sanger has made enormous strides in their lifetimes and in mine. But even today, sadly, there are those who would completely wreck all of their tireless work and deprive us all of our right to plan our families.

I am not talking about the people who conduct their own lives according to their own beliefs and do not try to impose their beliefs on the rest of us even if those beliefs forbid abortion or contraception. These are not the people who endanger our reproductive rights and privacy.

The ones who deeply worry me are the minority who do wish to force us all to live according to their rules. These few people are using whatever political power they can muster to destroy our freedom. We must oppose them — with the same courage with which my parents and Margaret Sanger opposed the moralistic repressionists of *their* day.

The world is a fascinating place. But it is filled with wild injustices that cry out to be rectified. That's what Planned Parenthood has been struggling to do, for three generations: to ensure a decent existence and a healthy, self-empowered life for every woman and man. I cherish the freedom of choice that has allowed me to shape my life. Why should *any* individual, *anywhere*, have anything less?

Katharine Hepburn

CONTENTS

75 YEARS OF CHOICE

Choice.

The word is nearly synonymous with the American dream.

It means the freedom to arrive by our own paths at our beliefs and moral values — to determine what we will say, what we will read and with whom we will associate — to elect our government representatives — to decide without interference how to conduct the personal, private aspects of our lives.

These liberties have been sacred to Americans since the founding of our democratic, pluralistic society.

But the right to choice in the most private matter of childbearing was not recognized for American women until the second half of the 20th century.

This freedom — described by a federal judge as "nearly allied to a woman's right to be"— was won only after generations of women had lost their health and lives to unplanned and unwanted childbearing. It was secured as the result of a struggle that first erupted into headlines 75 years ago, on October 16, 1916.

On that day, a former nurse named Margaret Sanger defied New York City law by opening a "clinic"— actually, a center for contraceptive instruction— in Brooklyn, New York.

The clinic remained open just 10 days. In that time Sanger, her sister Ethel Byrne, and fellow activist Fania Mindell provided birth control advice and counseling to hundreds of women who had nowhere else to turn. Many had eight or more children and were ill and old before their time. Several told Sanger that they were on the verge of suicide for fear of further childbearing.

The "birth control sisters" were ostracized, ridiculed and sentenced to jail for violating the laws against disseminating birth control information. But the movement they ignited soon led to the founding of grass-roots organizations across America, which fought determinedly for more enlightened attitudes, better methods of birth control and an end to anti-birth control laws. In 1939, these grass-roots organizations joined together, forming what initially was called the Birth Control Federation of America and eventually was named the Planned Parenthood Federation of America (PPFA).

Today Planned Parenthood is the nation's leading guardian of the tradition of choice established by those early struggles. Through a network of more than 900 centers in 49 states and the District of Columbia, it carries on the dual mission of service and advocacy that Margaret Sanger began long ago.

Planned Parenthood affiliates provide sexuality education and comprehensive reproductive health care to four million people annually. Their services range from birth control to cancer screening, treatment of sexually transmitted diseases, abortion services, infertility counseling and prenatal care. PPFA's international division serves women and men in the developing nations of Asia, Africa and Latin America.

For the past 75 years, the Planned Parenthood movement's visible, unflinching leadership has expanded the frontiers of reproductive freedom and extended the tradition of choice to new generations.

But while we appreciate how far we have come, we cannot lose sight of what remains to be done.

Ironically — just as in Margaret Sanger's day — American women today have fewer birth control options than their counterparts in western Europe. Even women in some developing countries have more birth control methods available to them than Americans.

Access to essential family planning information and services is denied to millions of women and men, in the U.S. and around the world. Without this access, choice is a mere abstraction.

In part because of the inadequacy of current methods and restrictions on access, more than three million American women experience unwanted pregnancies every year.

Nearly half of them end in abortion.

Almost one million of these unwanted pregnancies occur to teens— a rate of teen pregnancy that exceeds that of most other countries in the developed world.

Meanwhile, a small but strident anti-family planning minority— the descendants of those who opposed the early birth control pioneers— are determined to turn back advances in reproductive health and reproductive rights and drive women back to the perils of the late 19th and early 20th centuries.

For 75 years, Planned Parenthood and the American people have fought to defeat sexual and reproductive bigotry and ignorance. The oppression, suffering and despair that catapulted Margaret Sanger's movement have been overcome by the establishment of the right to choose when and whether to bear children. The pictures and stories in this volume are the mementos of those remarkable people of the birth control movement and their achievements.

But the courage, vision and struggle celebrated here are more than part of a glorious past. They are vital to the present and future, as the Planned Parenthood Federation nationwide extends this tradition into the next millennium.

THE 1910s: A TRADITION BEGINS

"I'm a police officer. You're under arrest."

—Margaret Whitehurst, member of the New York City vice squad,
to Margaret Sanger, October 26, 1916

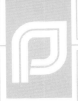

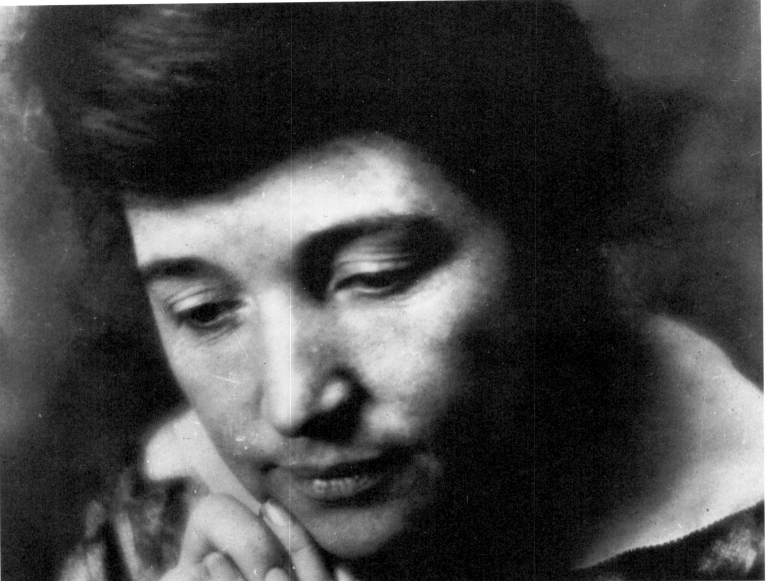

Margaret Sanger (1879-1966)

The 1910s were a time of cultural, political and social ferment. Social critics lamented the demise of the traditional family. Women in increasing numbers worked outside the home, principally in low-paid factory and sweatshop jobs. Intellectuals debated socialism, while radical labor leaders demanded a shorter work week. Women marched for suffrage. Provocative new styles in music and painting challenged convention in the arts.

In this climate, progressive thinkers inevitably began to question the late 19th-century Comstock laws that forbade contraception as well as abortion as forms of "obscenity." Among those who spoke out

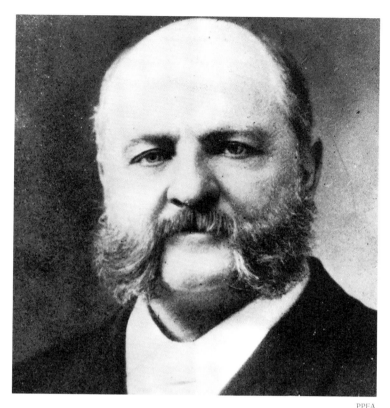

Anthony Comstock (1844-1915) was a self-appointed anti-vice crusader from New York, who in the 1870s managed to shepherd through Congress a stringent anti-obscenity statute. This statute forbade, among other "impurities," the importing or mailing of contraceptives or contraceptive information. In the same era, Comstock-type statutes enacted in many state legislatures forbade the dissemination or, in some cases, even the use of contraceptives. Comstock was so zealous and effective in the enforcement of these laws that by the late 19th century, the subject of contraception had become unmentionable — even in major medical textbooks.

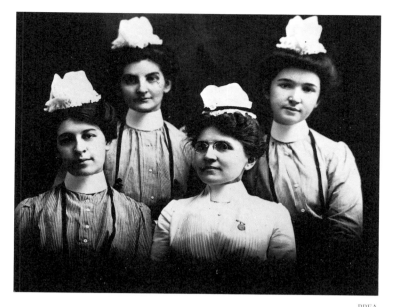

Margaret Sanger (right) on her graduation from the nursing school of White Plains (New York) Hospital

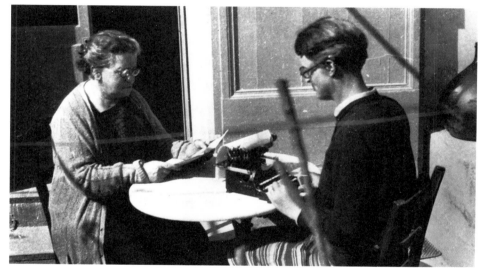

Emma Goldman (1869-1940) fought in the 1910s, like Sanger, for women's right to practice contraception. She and her partner, Ben Reitman, were jailed several times for speeches judged in violation of Comstock laws. She is shown here at left dictating her memoirs.

publicly and forcefully against involuntary motherhood were Emma Goldman, the socialist leader, and Mary Ware Dennett, a well-known suffragist. But none was more single-minded, persuasive or effective than a young woman named Margaret Sanger.

The sixth of 11 children in a poor Irish family, Sanger had seen her own mother die at the age of 49 as the result of tuberculosis contracted after too many pregnancies. In the early 1910s, she was working as a maternity nurse on the Lower East Side of New York, delivering babies in the homes of poor, mostly immigrant women. The women Sanger nursed knew nothing of how to prevent pregnancy and, because of the Comstock laws, could get no information from their doctors. Instead, they resorted to the illegal practitioners of five-dollar abortions, on whose tables many of them died.

"Tales," Sanger wrote, "were poured into my ears — a baby born dead, great relief — the death of an older child, sorrow but again relief of a sort — the story told a thousand times of death from abortion and children going into institutions. I shuddered with horror as I listened to the details and studied the reasons back of them — destitution linked with excessive childbearing. The waste of life seemed utterly senseless."

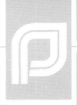

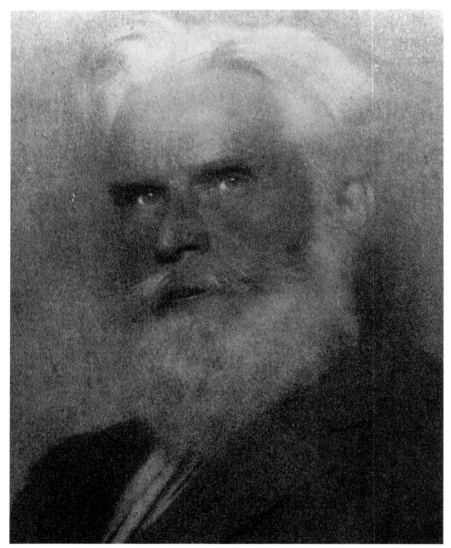

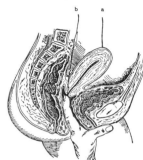

Pages from Margaret Sanger's booklet on contraception, "Family Limitation" (1915), with pictures of a French pessary (a precursor of the diaphragm) on the left and female reproductive organs on the right.

Havelock Ellis (1859-1939), author of the encyclopedic Studies in the Psychology of Sex, was one of the first writers to document the universality and variety of human sexuality. A close friend of Margaret Sanger from the time they met in England in 1915, he greatly influenced Sanger's perspective on sexual expression as normal and healthy.

One day in 1912, Sanger saw a patient named Sadie Sachs come close to death from a botched illegal abortion. When Sachs begged her doctor to tell her how not to get pregnant, he laughed and responded genially, "You can't have your cake and eat it too. Tell Jake to sleep on the roof." Three months later, Sanger was called again to the Sachs's home — in time to witness her patient's death, apparently from another illegal abortion. At that point, Sanger vowed to devote herself to a movement to free women from unwanted pregnancy and childbearing.

To educate herself for the battle, Sanger traveled to Europe to find out how women on that continent prevented conception. There she came upon recipes for contraceptive douches, tampons and suppositories and learned of the use of rubber pessaries (later called diaphragms) to prevent pregnancy. Sanger returned to New York determined to spread the word about these lifesaving measures. She coined the phrase "birth control," started publishing a newspaper called *The Woman Rebel* and wrote a pamphlet, "Family Limitation," that explained in simple, nonclinical language the preparation and use of European-style contraceptives.

In 1914, the federal government indicted Sanger for nine separate violations of the Comstock law arising from alleged obscenity in *The Woman Rebel*. In her reluctance to face trial, she fled back to Europe, where she spent the better part of a year advancing her knowledge of contraception. She was particularly impressed by her visits to the Dutch contraceptive clinics run by Dr. Johannes Rutgers, which prescribed comfortable, easy-to-insert diaphragms with

PPFA

EW WOMAN'S PAPER HELD UP AS OBSCENE

ncle Sam Won't Stand for Mrs. Sanger's Remarks on Keeping Families Down.

Deputy Attorney-General W. H. La-ar has declared in Washington that "he Woman Rebel," a monthly pa-r published in this city, which has ist made its initial bow to "an ad-anced thinking, frankly speaking minine clientele," is obscene and un-ailable at the New York Post-Office any other post-office. The New ork Post-Office was notified of the ecision yesterday and acted at once. In Mr. Lamur's opinion this paper so is incendiary literature. The aper has for its motto:

"No Gods; no masters."

One of the articles is by Mrs. Mar-aret Sanger of No. 34 Post avenue, ho is editor and proprietor of the ublication. She deals with what ight be termed the voluntary dimin-hing of the size of families of the oor. She advocates the dissemina-on of scientific information among oor women and says:

"A law forbids the imparting of in-rmation on this subject, the penalty ing several years' imprisonment. . it not time to defy the law? What tter place could be found than in the ages of the Woman Rebel?"

In a leading article is stated:

"An early feature will be a series articles written by the editor for irls from fourteen to eighteen years age. In the present chaos of sex mosphere it is difficult for the girl this uncertain age to know what do or what really constitutes clean ving without prudishness."

This article ridicules "white slav-ry," drugged drink stories and the ike, and then declares that it ex-ects to "circulate among women of he underworld. These women are ked to voice their opinions in the Woman Rebel and expose police who ersecute them.

"A Woman's Duty" is described hus!

"To look the world in the face with a go-to-hell look in the eyes; to have an ideal; to speak and act in defiance of convention."

oman Rebel claims the right to be azy; the right to be an unmarried nother; the right to destroy; the ight to create; the right to love; the ight to live."

Emma Goldman is one of the con-ributors. Others whose names are sted to articles are Voltairine De leyre, Teresa Billington, Greig, orothy Kelly, Elizabeth Kleen, atherine Holt, J. Edward Morgan nd Marion Howard.

Mrs. Sanger was notified yesterday...

THE WOMAN REBEL

NO GODS NO MASTERS

ORK CALL—TUESDAY, OCT...

WOMAN REBEL EDITOR ON TRIAL

Margaret H. Sanger, Radical Writer, May Be Placed on Trial Today.

Margaret H. Sanger, editor of the Woman Rebel, will be placed on trial today in United States District Court, room 331, Postoffice Building, provid-ed a case begun yesterday is cleared off the calendar. Mrs. Sanger is charged with sending "obscene and indecent" matter through the mail. Simon H. Pollock, her attorney, and many radicals were in the courtroom all of yesterday waiting for the case to be called.

There are four counts in the in-dictment against Mrs. Sanger. The charges allege "indecency" because of editorial articles written by Mrs. San-ger, in which she is alleged to have advocated birth control.

A strong defense committee is being organized for the purpose of protect-ing Mrs. Sanger from being railroad-ed to prison on what is generally con-sidered to be a ridiculous charge.

Unjust, Says Mrs. Boissevain.

Mrs. Ines Milholland Boissevain, well known suffragist, when seen by a reporter for The Call yesterday, came out boldly for Mrs. Sanger, saying that a great injustice would be done the defendant should she be con-victed.

"This is a question of common sense," said Mrs. Boissevain, who is a lawyer. "A little common sense ought to convince any one that Mrs. Sanger does not come within the meaning of the statute against inde-cency and obscenity. This statute was intended to make it unlawful to mail pictures without serious purpose, but of a suggestive nature. I refer to the pictures and jokes of the boule-vard type.

"But Mrs. Sanger is a serious...

reason it is wrong to say that she has violated the statute. The statute was not drawn up for such a case. This, it appears to me, is plain common sense.

"This case should be brought to the attention of the public. I be-lieve that birth control is a legiti-mate subject for serious discussion, and for this reason the intelligent women of New York should do some-thing.

Plain Talks for Plain People.

"Medical journals discuss birth control. But the writers in these scientific journals couch their ideas in language that is above the head of the average person. It appears as though Mrs. Sanger wrote on the same subject, only she talked plain English that could be understood by plain people, so she has been in-dicted.

In addition to the charge of "in-decency," Mrs. Sanger is alleged to have published a short article which advocated violence. This constitutes the fourth count and will serve to complicate the case, it is said.

Friends of Mrs. Sanger say that the governments of Europe make no effort to suppress discussion of birth control.

WOMAN REBEL'S EDITOR ARRESTED ON P. O. ORDER

Three Indictments Against Mrs. Sanger—Charge Ad-vocacy of Murder.

Not content with holding up three is-sues of the Woman Rebel, a monthly journal dedicated to the emancipation of woman, the United States postal authori-ties yesterday caused Mrs. Margaret H. Sanger, its editor, to be arraigned on three indictments charging violation of postal laws. The authorities allege ad-vocacy of "assassination and the use of dynamite in social reform."

In the two other indictments Mrs. Sanger is charged with publishing "ob-scene, vile and indecent" articles con-cerning sex matters. Mrs. Sanger en-tered a temporary plea of not guilty be-...

marily at the instigation of Anthony Comstock.

A protest against the refusal to mail the papers was made by the editor and nothing was heard until yesterday. As Mrs. Sanger was at her home, 34 Post avenue, the Bronx, preparing another is-sue, she was notified by the authorities of the indictments and immediately surren-dered herself.

"This had to come sooner or later," she said later, "and I welcome any method of vindicating my theories. Until the postal laws are changed in certain re-gards, it will be impossible for me to carry out the great work I have started for my sex."

WINS FIGHT FOR BIRTH CONTROL

Case Against Mrs. Sanger Thrown Out of Court With-out a Hearing.

Mrs. Margaret Sanger is not to be tried by the United States Government on the indictment found against her in August, 1914, for sending information about birth control through the mails.

Assistant Federal Attorney Content obtained dismissal of the indictment by Judge Dayton, to the surprise of Mrs. Sanger, who had insistently de-manded opportunity to vindicate her-self and her cause in court.

Mr. Content presented a memoran-dum signed by District-Attorney Marshall, which stated that Mrs. San-ger was not a disorderly person, and while the Government believed the magazine articles in question un-mailable, there was a reasonable doubt. Besides, for two years she had made no attempt to repeat the alleged offense.

On the strength of these arguments Judge Dayton quashed the indict-ments. Mrs. Sanger then found her-self in the peculiar position of having escaped so much as a trial for writing and sending through the mails litera-ture that caused her husband, William Sanger, to be sentenced to thirty days in jail for the simple act of handing one of the offending documents to a visitor at his office.

Mrs. Sanger, informed that the pro-ceedings had been dropped, called the outcome "a splendid triumph."

Miss Helen Todd telephoned the newspapers that the Sanger Commit-tee, organized for the defense of the accused woman, would hold a jubilee...

THE BIRTH CONTROL REVIEW

Dedicated to the Principle of Intelligent and Voluntary Motherhood

Volume One — FEBRUARY 1917 — Number One

SHALL WE BREAK THIS LAW?

By MARGARET SANGER

Fifteen cents a copy — *One dollar a year*

PPFA

Sanger began publishing the Birth Control Review in 1917, while she was awaiting trial for her role in the Brownsville clinic. It became the leading voice of the movement she helped found from then until 1930, when it ceased publication.

Margaret Sanger's first trip to Europe inspired her with a vision of what women could achieve, once freed from enforced motherhood. On her return, she began to publish a radical journal, The Woman Rebel, which was soon declared unmail-able under the federal Comstock law.

spring rims designed by the pioneering gynecologist Aletta Jacobs. Armed with new knowledge and confidence, in mid-1915, Sanger gathered her courage and returned to the U.S. to face trial.

By the time she returned, the birth control cause was gathering popular support, and Sanger herself — a mother of three, attractive, soft-spoken and convincing — proved to be a highly sympathetic public figure. Embarrassed at the growing adulation for her, the government dropped the indict-ment. Sanger, riding a wave of popularity, embarked on the first of many speaking tours to promote reproductive choice, lecturing in towns from New Rochelle, New York, to Spokane, Washington. She was quietly led in and out of halls through freight entrances, faced down hostile audiences, endured hecklers and spent several nights in jails for her outspokenness. In one city after another, she inspired courageous volunteers to create advocacy organizations to fight for birth control — several of them the predecessors of today's Planned Parenthood affiliates.

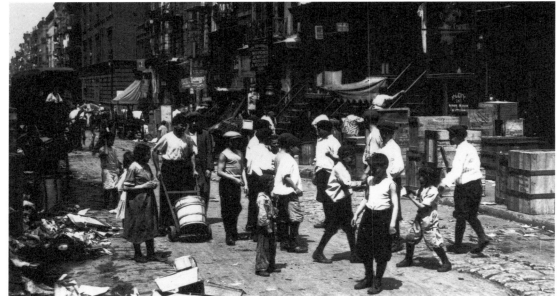

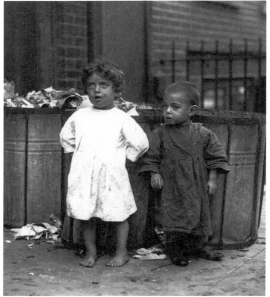

Children from New York's Lower East Side whom Margaret Sanger might have seen when she began her work as a nurse

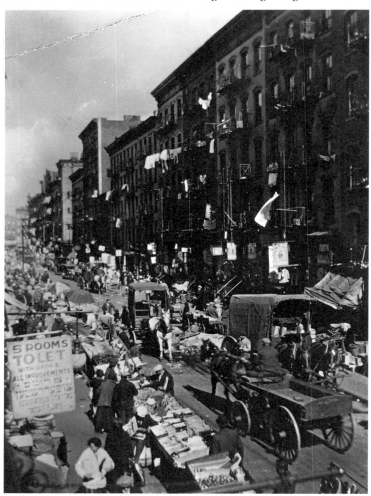

The street in Brownsville, Brooklyn, where Margaret Sanger opened her first clinic

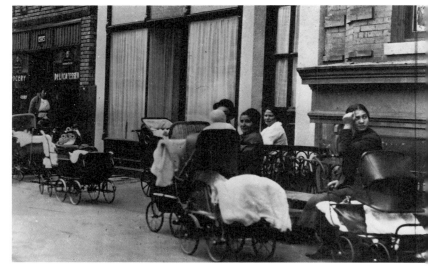

Women form a line outside America's first birth control clinic.

In 1916, encouraged by the success of her first nationwide tour, Sanger decided it was time to move beyond writing and speaking and into direct action. She determined to open a storefront office in New York City that would provide contraceptive advice and counseling directly to women who needed those services.

With Fania Mindell, a devoted supporter she had met during a lecture in Chicago, Sanger toured the poor immigrant neighborhood of Brownsville, Brooklyn, until she located suitable quarters for her center at 46 Amboy Street. After recruiting her sister, Ethel Byrne, a licensed nurse, to help, she opened the "clinic" for business on October 16, 1916.

Planned Parenthood League of Massachusetts

In 1917, Boston police arrested a young radical named Van Kleek Allison for distributing pamphlets about contraception to Boston factory workers. Allison was convicted and sentenced to a term of three years — but not before outraged citizens had founded the Birth Control League of Massachusetts (predecessor of the Planned Parenthood League of Massachusetts) to defend him and promote support for reproductive freedom. The Massachusetts fight went on nearly 50 years, until finally, in 1966, the state legislature passed a law permitting contraceptive services for married couples.

The women and families began lining up before the doors even opened. Mindell provided child care while Sanger and Byrne addressed the women and husbands in a rear room, explaining contraception, distributing copies of "Family Limitation," and referring the women to local pharmacies that Sanger had made sure would have plenty of pessaries on hand. (Though illegal for contraceptive purposes, pessaries were familiar to American doctors and pharmacists as treatment for a prolapsed uterus or for the application of other medications.) At 7 p.m., the families, who paid 10 cents each for the service, were still coming. "A hundred women and 40 men passed through the doors, but we could not begin to finish the line," Sanger wrote. "The rest were told to return 'tomorrow.'"

The clinic was closed by the police on its tenth day, after providing advice and counseling to just 488 grateful women and men. The effort cost Sanger and the others many anxious, fearful days in court and ultimately led to 30-day jail sentences for Sanger and Byrne. But that pioneering effort pointed the way for generations of Planned Parenthood activists to come and changed the map of reproductive rights forever.

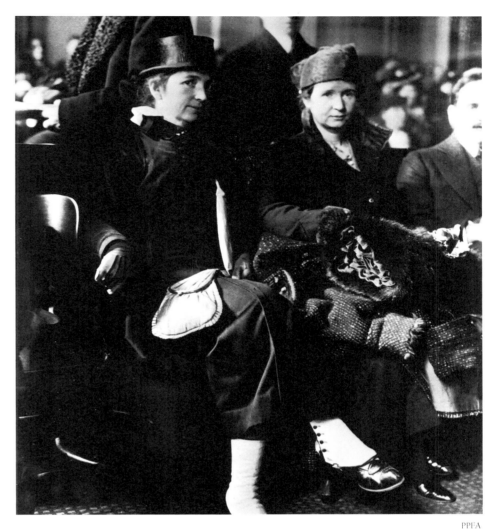

PPFA

Sanger and her sister, Ethel Byrne, on trial in criminal court in New York. Sentenced to 30 days in jail, Byrne went on a hunger strike and nearly died, after becoming the first woman in a U.S. prison to be force-fed through a tube.

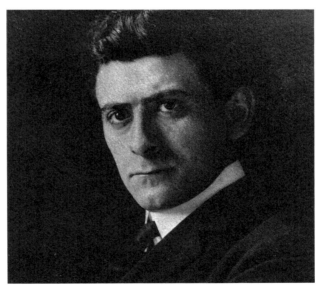

Sophia Smith Collection, Smith College

William Sanger, an architect and Sanger's first husband, became a hero of the birth control movement when he was indicted for giving a copy of "Family Limitation" to an undercover agent posing as a desperate father and husband. Sentenced to a fine of $150 or 30 days in jail, he made headlines by telling the judge, "I would rather be in jail with my self-respect than in your place without it."

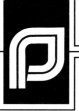

THE 1920s: MAKING HEADWAY

"The doctor told me I was too weak to have children. He doesn't want me to have any for a while but what shall I do? He won't tell me how not to have any. So I thought I would ask you if you know of any way....Please try to help me if you can. I would be ever so thankful and I am asking only for the sake of these little ones so that I can bring them up halfway decent."

—Letter received by the American Birth Control League in the 1920s and reprinted in *Motherhood in Bondage* (1928)

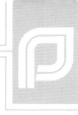

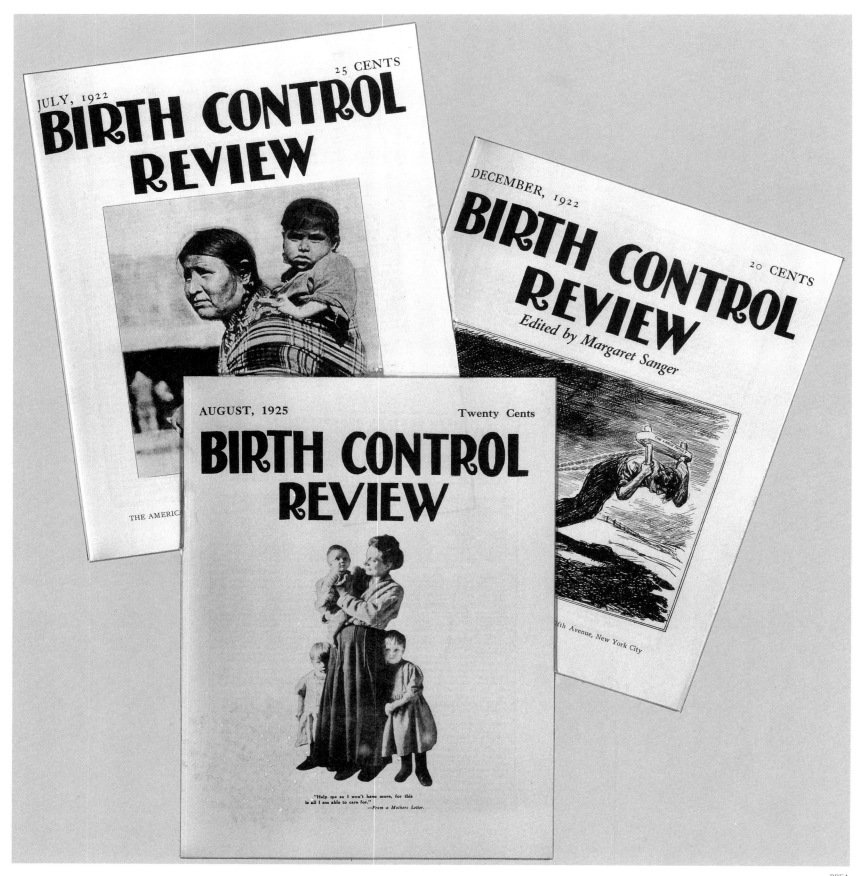

As these illustrations show, the covers of the Birth Control Review appealed to readers' sympathy for women overburdened by poverty and childrearing. The content of the journal, however, was wide-ranging and scholarly, as Sanger sought to demonstrate support for the birth control cause by publishing the articles of leading intellectuals in many fields.

Among those whose work Sanger published occasionally were the so-called eugenicists, a powerful and influential movement of the time. The eugenicists argued that, for the sake of what they called "race betterment," wealthy and educated people were morally obligated to have large families. They often opposed the use of birth control because they felt the rich would use it and the poor would not. While Sanger cooperated with the eugenics movement, in the belief that its popularity lent respectability to her cause, she also clearly stated her disagreement with its views, emphasizing "the necessity of leaving the decision as to the number of children and the time of their arrival to the mother, whether she be rich or poor."

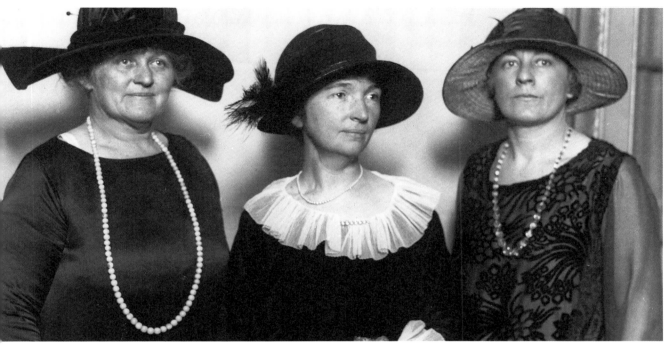

Sanger stands between two other women who played major roles in the birth control movement in the 1920s: Dr. Dorothy Bocker (left) and Anne Kennedy (right). Kennedy, a longtime close associate of Sanger's, was an editor of the Birth Control Review *and a chief organizer of the American Birth Control League. Bocker was the first physician whom Sanger hired to run the Birth Control Clinical Research Bureau when it opened in 1923. Although Bocker's only previous experience, working for the public health service in Georgia, had little relevance to prescribing birth control, she was the only doctor Sanger could persuade to risk her license by running the pioneering clinic. In 1924, Bocker was succeeded by Dr. Hannah Stone, who remained at the helm of the clinic until her death in 1941.*

UPI

The end of World War I hammered the last nail in the coffin of Victorian ideals. During the "roaring '20s," the ferment that characterized intellectual circles in the previous decade spread to an entire generation. Regardless of its impact on the use of alcohol, Prohibition certainly led to disrespect for laws that contradicted prevailing attitudes. Women won the vote, and while universal suffrage failed to produce the egalitarian society some had anticipated, it added to the sense of freedom and independence that many middle-class women felt.

Most women, however, continued to struggle against overwhelming burdens. Massive immigration swelled the populations of American cities with poor families, who lived in crowded tenements in conditions that fostered disease and early death. Although the Comstock laws remained in force and conservative groups (including the medical profession) continued to oppose any "artificial" prevention of pregnancy, the tragic circumstances of these families lent force and credibility to the arguments for birth control.

In 1921, Margaret Sanger, with the help of funds from many supporters worldwide,

launched an organization called the American Birth Control League (ABCL), with headquarters at 104 Fifth Avenue in New York. Its purpose was to win greater public support for birth control by demonstrating the close connection between a woman's ability to limit her fertility and such other great issues as war, famine and public health. Sanger also defied the morality of the times by declaring that women had the right to experience sexual pleasure and that freeing them from the fear of pregnancy would help to achieve that.

In 1928, Sanger left the ABCL, but it continued to advocate nationally for reproductive rights under the leadership of Ellen Dwight-Jones and others. During the first four years of the ABCL's existence, Sanger received more than a million letters from desperate women requesting information about contraception. From 1923, Sanger employed a staff of three to seven just to answer the mail. Eventually, she published several hundred of the most powerful letters in a book called *Motherhood in Bondage* that did much to increase public sympathy and understanding of the need for birth control.

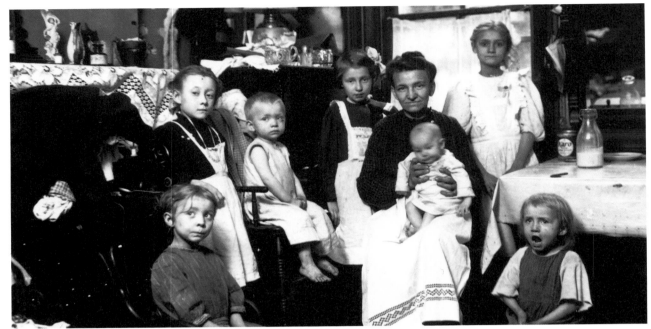

Women who worked from dawn until night to support large families on meager incomes were typical of the clients of the early birth control clinics.

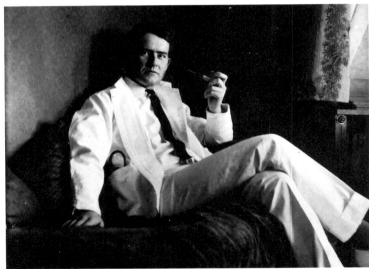

Dr. Thomas Hepburn (above), father of the actress, Katharine Hepburn, was one member of the medical profession who gave strong, early support to the birth control movement.

Katharine Houghton Hepburn (above right), mother of the actress, was a close ally of Margaret Sanger and one of the founders of the Connecticut Birth Control League.

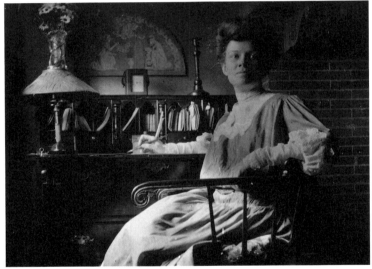

In 1923, with the help of a contribution from a private donor she had met in England, Sanger rented a room next to the league's office, where she established the nation's first true birth control clinic — this one under a physician's supervision. She called this new enterprise the Birth Control Clinical Research Bureau, a name it retained until 1940, when it became the Margaret Sanger Research Bureau. (In 1973, the research bureau dissolved and transferred its assets to Planned Parenthood of New York City, where the Margaret Sanger Center continues to provide reproductive health care services and to conduct research.)

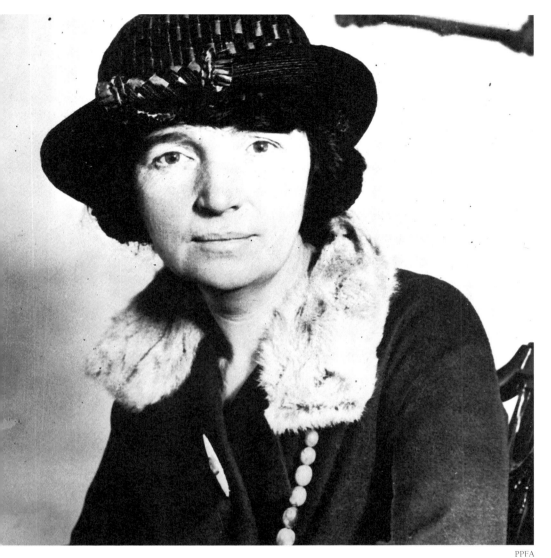

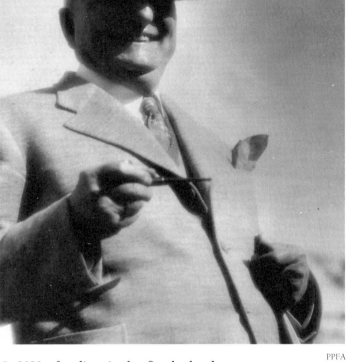

In 1921, after divorcing her first husband, Sanger married Noah Slee (1861-1943), a wealthy widower who was the president of Three-in-One Oil. Slee remained a generous backer of the birth control movement until his death.

Sanger's passionate interest in the liberation of women worldwide began early in her career. In the 1920s, she traveled to Japan, China, India and the Soviet Union, where she lectured and tried to persuade government leaders and intellectuals to support birth control efforts. This portrait was taken in March 1922 in San Francisco, her point of embarkation to Japan, where her speaking tour coincided with tours by Albert Einstein, Bertrand Russell and H.G. Wells.

Unlike the Brownsville center, the clinical research bureau conformed to the letter of New York's Comstock law, which allowed physicians to prescribe contraception "for the prevention of disease." The original intent of this law was simply to allow men to use condoms when they frequented prostitutes. Sanger's clinical research bureau set out to prove that making contraception available to women was also vital to "preventing disease" — once disease was defined broadly enough to embrace the ill health and economic stress brought on by unwanted childbearing.

Dr. Hannah Stone, a Russian-born gynecologist and obstetrician who became known to thousands of her patients as the "madonna of birth control," was the clinic's director from 1924 until her death in 1941, when her husband, Dr. Abraham Stone, took over. Hannah Stone suffered professional ostracism and public humiliation for her association with Sanger and with birth control. She lost her connection with Lying-In Hospital and for years was denied membership in the New York County Medical Society. In 1929, she was arrested in a brutal police raid on the clinic, apparently instigated by a complaint from the Catholic church. Yet her work was of critical importance.

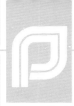

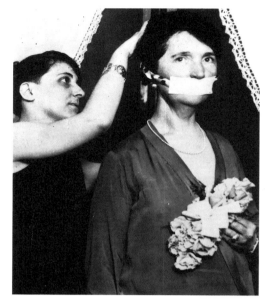

Sanger was often prevented by opposition from the Catholic church hierarchy from speaking in public. Here, in April 1929, after Boston authorities threatened to bar her from the stage of Ford Hall Forum, she appeared in a gag while Arthur M. Schlesinger, Sr., read her speech.

An even more infamous effort to silence the movement took place on November 14, 1921, at New York City's Town Hall. Sanger had called a well-publicized mass meeting to announce the formation of the American Birth Control League — but when she arrived with the keynote speaker, Harold Cox, editor of the Edinburgh Review, she found the doors locked and 100 uniformed police ringing the hall. Sanger attempted to speak anyway and was arrested for disorderly conduct. Meanwhile, the meeting's organizers learned that the police had taken their orders from the Catholic archdiocese. This outrageous violation of free speech had the effect of rallying sympathizers to the birth control movement and swelling the ranks of the new league.

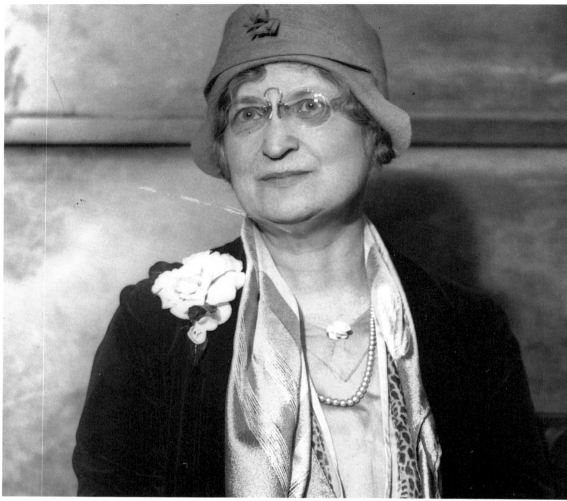

A prominent suffragist and early activist for birth control, Mary Ware Dennett (1872-1947) headed the Voluntary Parenthood League, which sought to legalize birth control in the 1920s by lobbying for an act of Congress.

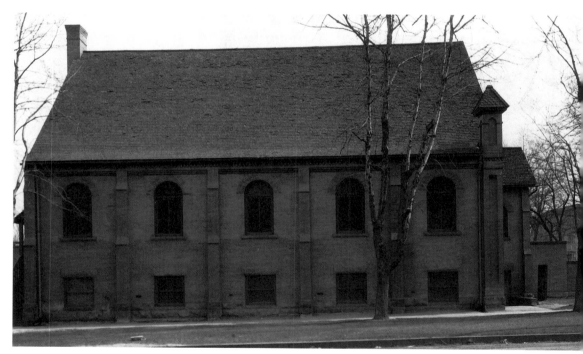

The church where Planned Parenthood of the Rocky Mountains (Colorado) was founded in 1926

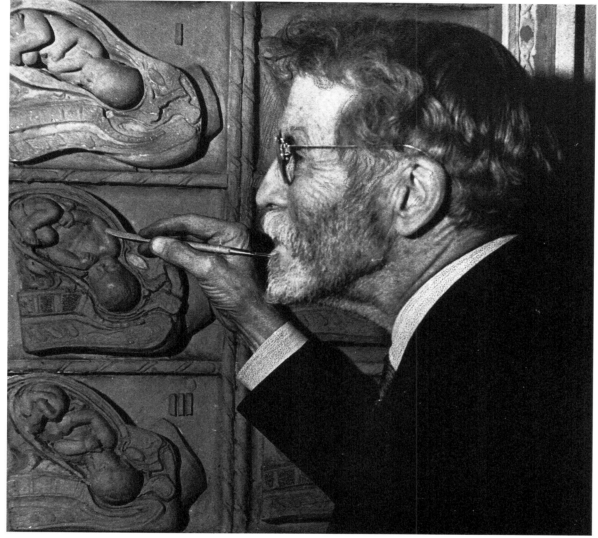

Dr. Robert Latou Dickinson (1861-1950), a pioneering sex researcher and one of the most eminent gynecologists of his day, played a vital role in convincing his profession that the practice of birth control was medically sound. An early champion of women's right to freedom from unwanted childbearing, he lent his support to the work of the Birth Control Clinical Research Bureau at a time when Sanger and Hannah Stone were shunned by most members of the medical profession. He was instrumental in persuading the editors of the Medical Journal and Record to publish Stone's early findings, and he rallied the medical profession to condemn the police raid on the research bureau in 1929. A noted sculptor, he also designed the medallion that was later presented as the PPFA Lasker Award.

Stone documented case histories of more than a thousand patients, showing not only the medical indications for prescribing contraception, but also circumstances such as low family income and poor living conditions that argued for the practice of birth control. Many of her cases included follow-up by a social worker, allowing comparisons between the well-being of women who received and used contraceptive methods and those who did not. This research played an essential role in establishing the impact of contraception on maternal health and in securing the support of the medical profession.

Inspired by the example of Sanger and Stone, birth control advocates across the country started clinics in their own communities. Denver activists, for instance,

began a shoestring operation in 1926 — forerunner of today's Planned Parenthood of the Rocky Mountains, which by 1990 was serving nearly 60,000 individuals a year.

Operating just once a week in a borrowed room in a church, the original Denver clinic had almost no money and was run by the efforts of volunteers: Mrs. T.D. Cunningham, Mrs. Imogene Daly Genter, Mrs. Montgomery Dorsey, Mrs. Charles Kassler, Mrs. Verner Reed, Mrs. James Rae Arneill, Mrs. V.L. Board. They arose at 6 a.m. to escort poor women to the clinic and care for their families, which typically included 12 or more children. According to a 1979 account, "Only loyalty, courage and imagination kept the idea and work afloat because these women encountered continual opposition and ridicule."

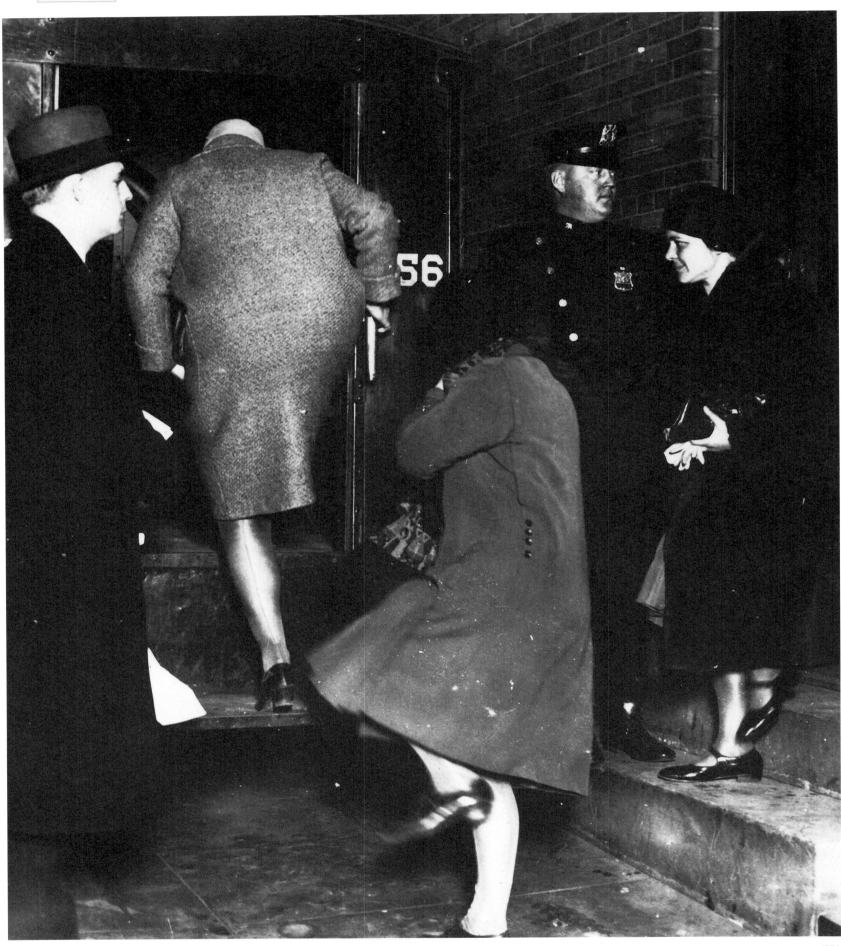

PPFA

April 15, 1929. Staff of the Birth Control Clinical Research Bureau are led into a paddy wagon after a police raid. Hannah Stone is in the doorway, at right.

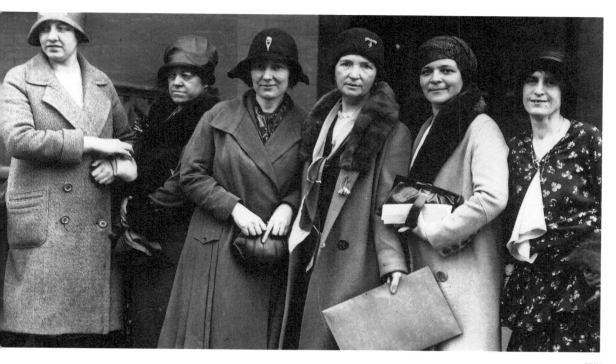

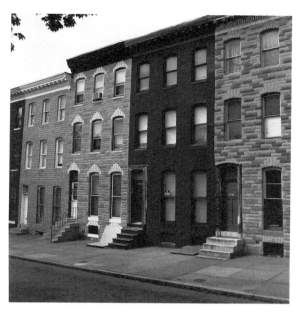

The block of brownstones in northeast Baltimore where Planned Parenthood of Maryland first opened for business in 1927

In this photo, taken shortly after the 1929 raid on the clinical research bureau, Margaret Sanger (fourth from left) stands between Dr. Elizabeth Pissoort (third from left) and Dr. Hannah Stone (second from right). The other women are nurses; their names are not known.

One year after the Denver clinic was founded, Dr. Bessie Moses, an obstetrician at Johns Hopkins Hospital in Baltimore, helped start Baltimore's Bureau of Contraceptive Advice (later, Planned Parenthood of Maryland) on the ground floor of a house in northeast Baltimore. The late Leonore Guttmacher, who became an honorary PPFA board member, recalled the volunteer work she did soon after the clinic opened:

"In those days the diaphragm was used almost exclusively. The patients were usually nervous, apprehensive that there might be a male doctor lurking about....This, despite the fact that most of our patients had had babies and male physicians had delivered them....Much of my job consisted of wiping perspiring faces with a cool, damp cloth, patting a clinging hand....Many spoke about fear of spoiling their 'nature' or their husband's 'pleasure' through using birth control. Some were afraid of losing their husbands. But they needed help so desperately they came to the clinic, despite the shame and the fear."

These halting steps into service delivery were crucial in establishing the tradition of choice. For once women had access, not just to the idea of birth control but to the means to practice it, they would never give up their freedom. And it was only a question of time before this access would be extended to many more.

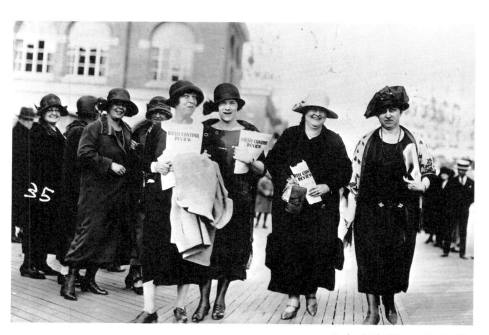

Volunteers sell the Birth Control Review on the streets of New York.

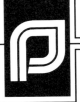

THE 1930s: VICTORY AND CONSOLIDATION

"The law process is a simple one; it is a matter of educating judges to the mores of the day."

—Morris Ernst, attorney for Margaret Sanger and the Birth Control Clinical Research Bureau

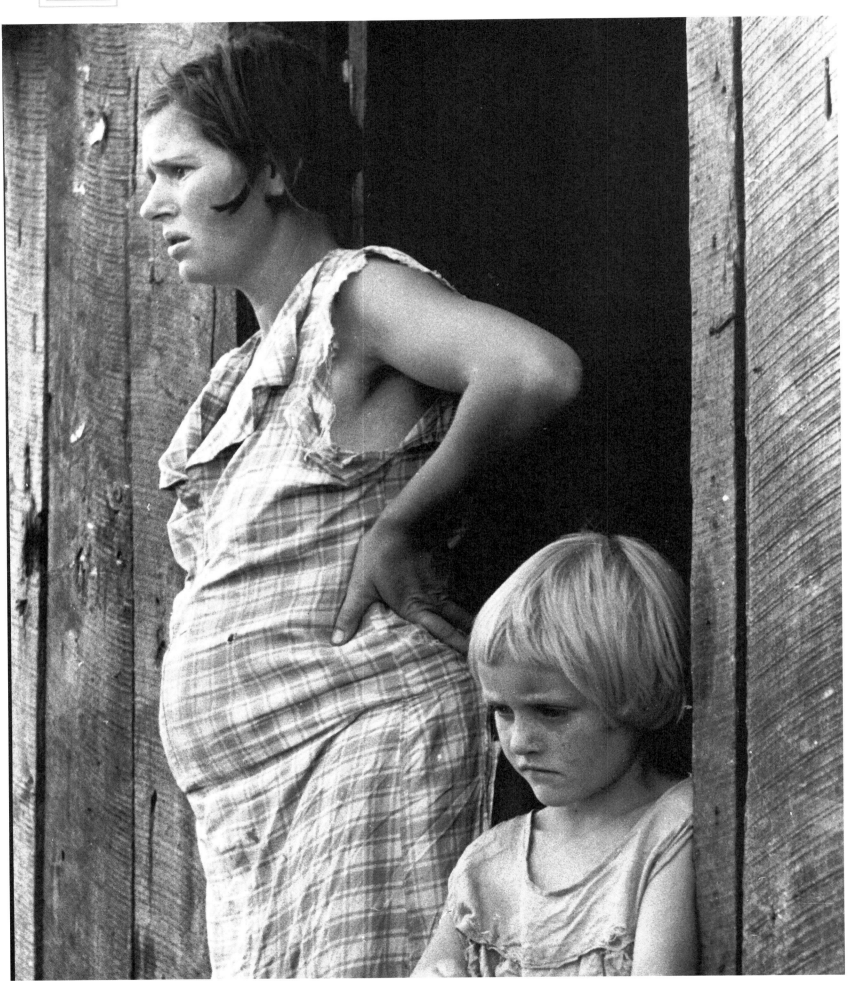

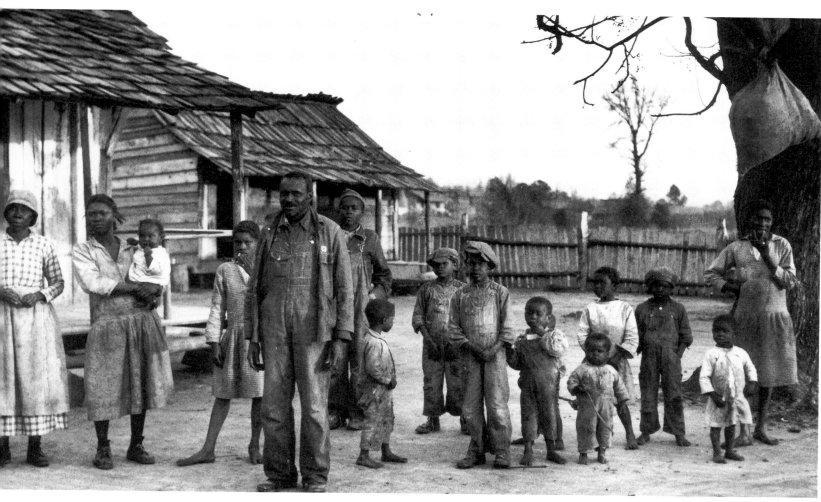

During the 1930s, as photos on these two pages show, business and farm failures led to starvation, and homeless families wandered the countryside.

The stock market crash of 1929 ushered in the worst economic disaster of American history. In the early 1930s, an estimated 25 percent of the labor force was unemployed. A million homeless people wandered the country. By the thousands, children starved. The Great Depression contributed to driving President Herbert Hoover out of office and paved the way for President Franklin Roosevelt's New Deal. As massive social welfare programs provided food, shelter and health care to desperate people, a new commitment to social justice took root in the hearts of Americans. In this climate, the birth control movement won new adherents and clinic services flourished — though often in the face of powerful minority opposition.

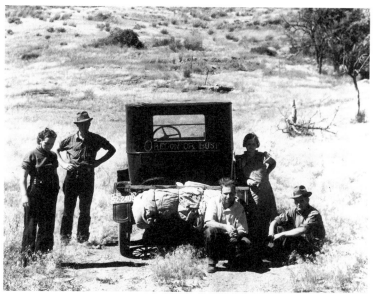

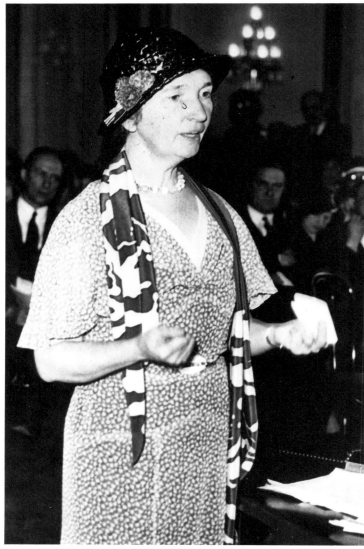

Underwood and Underwood

Margaret Sanger testifying before a Senate subcommittee as chair of the National Committee for Federal Legislation

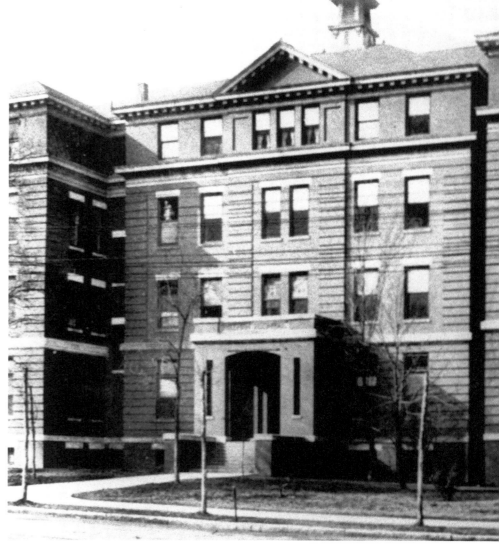

Univ. of Alabama/Birmingham, Medical Center Archives

Hillman Charity Hospital in Birmingham, Alabama, was the site of the first birth control clinic in the U.S. South, founded in 1930 as the Maternal Welfare Association of Jefferson County. It later became Planned Parenthood of Alabama and Mississippi, which is a major provider of women's health care in Alabama (where 35 of 67 counties have neither hospitals nor practicing gynecologists) and also one of the few providers of low-cost services in the state of Mississippi.

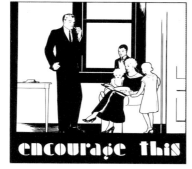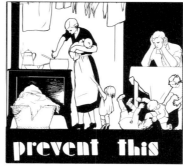

Worsinger Photo/PPFA

American Birth Control League poster. The predecessor of Planned Parenthood, the league worked to legalize birth control, served as a central clearinghouse for grass-roots birth control organizations and provided practical information and referrals to individual women.

In 1930, the South's first birth control clinic was founded in Birmingham, Alabama, by pediatrician Dr. Clifford Lamar and obstetrician Dr. Lee Turlington. After just three days, religious opponents had the clinic ousted from its original site in Hillman Charity Hospital. It reopened almost immediately in the waiting room of a public health tuberculosis clinic, where family planning patients were seen in the afternoon. The effort grew with the support of individual donors and contributions from such groups as the American Association of University Women, the Junior League, the National Council of

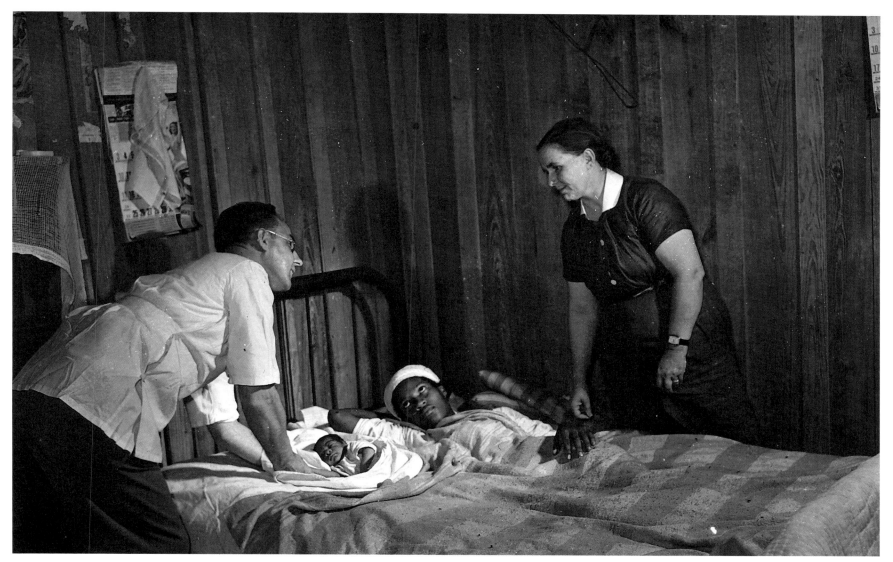

In the late 1930s, the extreme poverty and isolation of African-American families in the southern United States led several birth control organizations, under Margaret Sanger's leadership, to initiate the "Negro Project," designed to deliver birth control education and services to the rural South. The project had support from such prominent African-American leaders as W.E.B. DuBois, but was shelved with U.S. entry into World War II. This snapshot shows birth control field workers visiting a rural family at about the time the Negro Project was founded.

Jewish Women and the Episcopal Church, as well as, in the words of an official historian, "the quiet consent of public health authorities who recognized the need."

In 1935, in Dayton, Ohio, community leaders organized that area's first birth control clinic — forerunner of today's Planned Parenthood Association of Miami Valley. Twelve doctors served on the original medical advisory committee, on the condition that their involvement would receive no publicity. The clinic was held once weekly in the office of one of the doctors, Walter Ricketts. To

maintain their commitment to avoid publicity, board members recruited women by making personal visits to their homes.

"You should have seen us," wrote Susan Patterson, one of the first board members. "We had lists of prospective clients [furnished by schools and public health nurses] and went up one street and down the other, knocking on doors and urging people to at least come down to the clinic and see what it was all about. If anyone challenged us, we were engaged in 'protecting the health of these people, and family planning was a mere incidental.'"

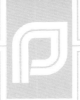

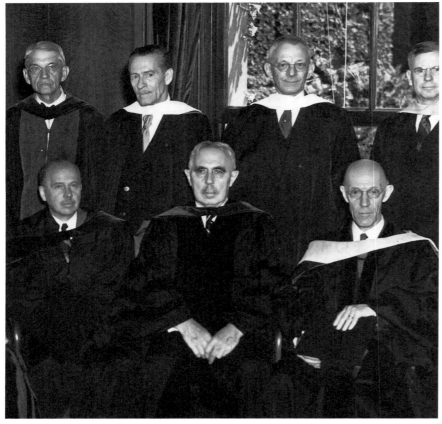

Judge Augustus Hand wrote the groundbreaking appeals court ruling in the case of *U.S. v. One Package of Japanese Pessaries.* He is shown here (seated, center), receiving an honorary degree from Yale University in 1939.

UPI/Bettmann

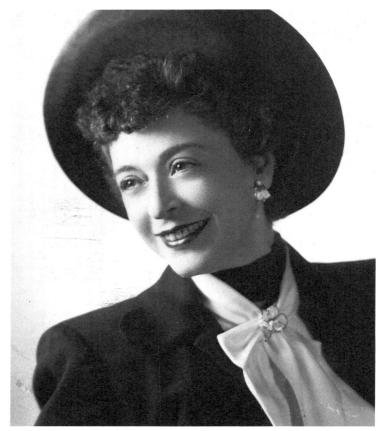

Collection of Irvin Schwartz

Harriet F. Pilpel (1911-1991)

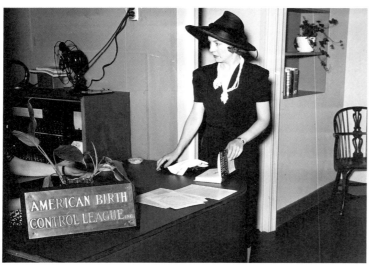

Zoltan S. Farkas/PPFA

A woman visits the American Birth Control League office at 104 Fifth Avenue in New York City.

Sanger herself spent the early 1930s in Washington, D.C., as head of an organization called the National Committee for Federal Legislation, which tried for five years to persuade Congress to revise the federal Comstock statute. While Congress refused to budge, a test case in federal court received a better reception.

The case had its origin in Sanger's interest in a new contraceptive device, a pessary designed by a Japanese physician. She ordered 120 of them to be shipped from Tokyo to Hannah Stone in New York. Since the federal Comstock law forbade, without exception, the importing of contraceptive devices, the shipment was seized and confiscated, laying the basis for the case with the unlikely name of *U.S. v. One Package of Japanese Pessaries.* It was argued by attorney Morris Ernst in federal district court in New York in 1935-1936.

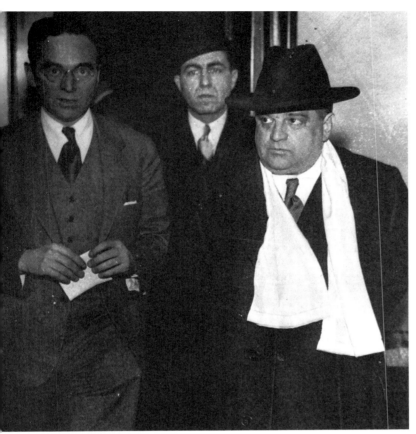

*Morris Ernst (left) with New York Mayor Fiorello LaGuardia. The
man behind them is unidentified.*

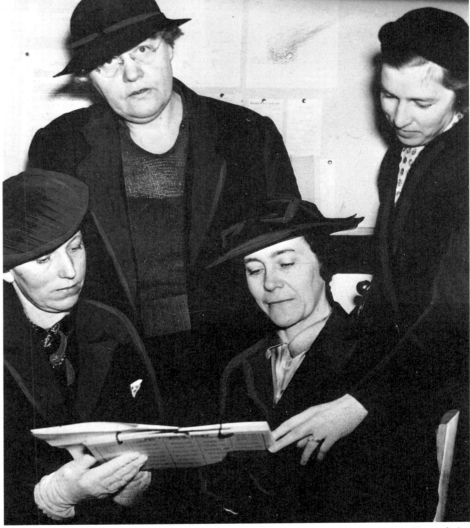

*Grass-roots leaders at a 1938 conference that helped lead to the merger of birth
control organizations throughout the country. Left to right are: Mrs. Carl
Waldron, Mrs. Charles Lundquist, Mrs. George Dunn, Mrs. Burton J. Case.*

On January 6, 1936, Judge Grover
Moskowitz declared that the government's
seizure of the pessaries stemmed from an
insupportably limited reading of the
Comstock statute. The government appealed.
Ernst, with the assistance of a young
Columbia University Law School graduate
named Harriet F. Pilpel, marshalled an
impressive body of evidence to argue the
appeal before a three-judge panel. Their brief
presented the extensive findings of Hannah
Stone and others to document the broad
impact of contraception on maternal health
and well-being. In the fall of 1936, Judge
Augustus Hand upheld the lower court ruling.
He stated that if Congress had had in the
1870s the same clinical data on the dangers of
pregnancy and the usefulness of contraception
that were available in the 1930s, it would
never have classified birth control as obscene.

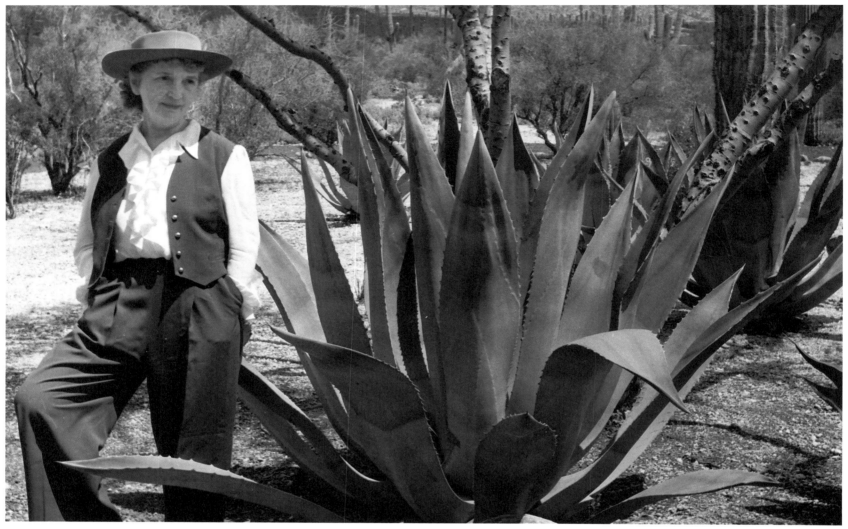

Margaret Sanger at her home in Tucson, Arizona, where she moved in the late 1930s

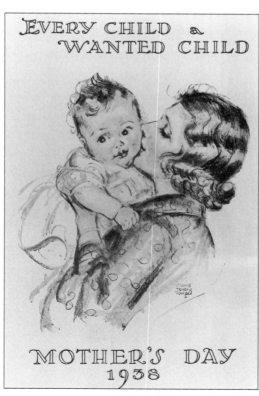

EVERY CHILD a
WANTED CHILD

*American Birth
Control League poster*

MOTHER'S DAY
1938

The application of the *One Package* decision was quite limited. It applied only to the importing of contraceptive devices from abroad by licensed physicians, and it had the force of law only in those states within the appellate court's jurisdiction. But because the court had acknowledged that birth control had both medical and socioeconomic significance, this ruling helped to solidify the tradition of choice. Its importance was underscored the following year, when the American Medical Association for the first time recognized contraception as a legitimate medical service and recommended its inclusion in medical school curricula.

In the same year, the state of North Carolina became the first to permit family

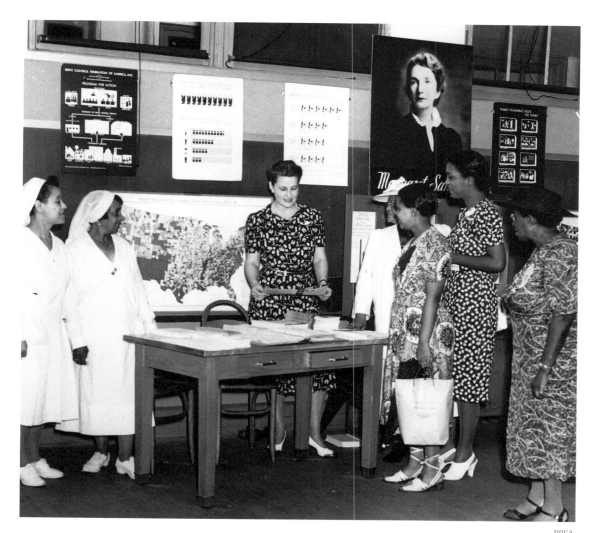

Health professionals attending a 1939 meeting of the National Medical Association in New York City gather at a table staffed by the newly founded Birth Control Federation of America.

PPFA

PPFA

Birth Control Information Through Public Health Clinics Favored in Survey

Carolina Clinic Plan Is Approved by Voters as Federation Meeting Opens

By DR. GEORGE GALLUP
Director, American Institute of Public Opinion

PRINCETON, N. J., Jan. 23.—With the adoption by South Carolina of a plan for birth control education as a regular part of its public health service, the American Institute of Public Opinion has conducted a survey to test public sentiment on extending this plan elsewhere.

This 1939 newsletter of the Birth Control Federation of America hailed the growing support of Americans for publicly funded birth control, as shown by a series of Gallup polls over the previous three years. By 1939, 77 percent of all Americans who had an opinion on the subject said that the government should make birth control information available to married couples who wanted it.

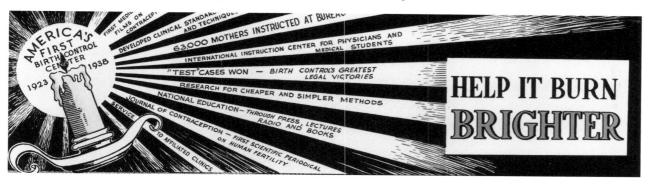

A poster honoring the 15th anniversary of the Birth Control Clinical Research Bureau, directed by Margaret Sanger

Sophia Smith Collection, Smith College

planning services to be offered as part of its public health program.

In June 1937, encouraged after a decade and a half of growth, the leaders of the American Birth Control League and the nation's hundreds of clinics came together to try to create a single, strong national organization. Constituting themselves as the Birth Control Council of America, they called in an outside consultant, Kenneth Rose of the John Price Jones fund raising and public relations agency, to advise them on the next steps. In January 1939, on a high tide of optimism, the movement's leaders announced the formation of the Birth Control Federation of America, with Margaret Sanger as honorary president and Kenneth Rose as acting director. In 1942, they would agree on a new name and become the Planned Parenthood Federation of America (PPFA).

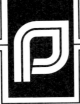

THE 1940s: EVERY WOMAN'S RIGHT

"I am writing to inquire the locations of birth control clinics located near here. Mrs. —— and I were married December 22nd during a furlough of mine....As an enlisted man I do not receive enough money to sustain a household by myself, let alone to have children. The only reason Mrs. —— and myself will be able to live together is her having a position as teacher in a nearby high school. During my service in the army I have had occasion several times to witness the utter despair of men, who trusted to hearsay methods of contraception, on learning that their wives were to have children."

—Letter reprinted in the PPFA newsletter, June 19, 1944

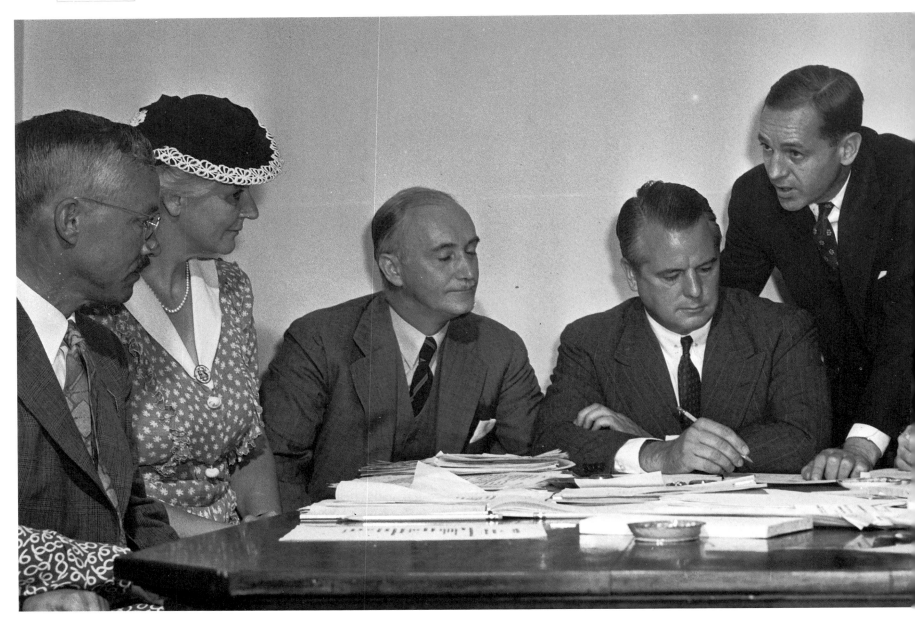

The PPFA board at the 1942 annual meeting, its first after the membership adopted the name Planned Parenthood Federation of America. The three men at the center are (left to right): Richard N. Pierson, M.D., chairperson of the Birth Control Federation of America (1939-1942); J.H.J. Upham, M.D., chairperson of PPFA (1942-1945) and Kenneth Rose, national director of PPFA (1939-1948).

World War II and its aftermath had a seismic impact on the nation's economic, cultural and social life. During the war, women enlisted in the "home-front army," taking over jobs in industry, agriculture and the professions that had never before been open to them. With men off to war and the future uncertain, many deferred raising families until peacetime.

Meanwhile, though, popular wisdom claimed that the declining birth rate in the U.S. had weakened the country internationally. "Pronatalists" stepped up their rhetoric after

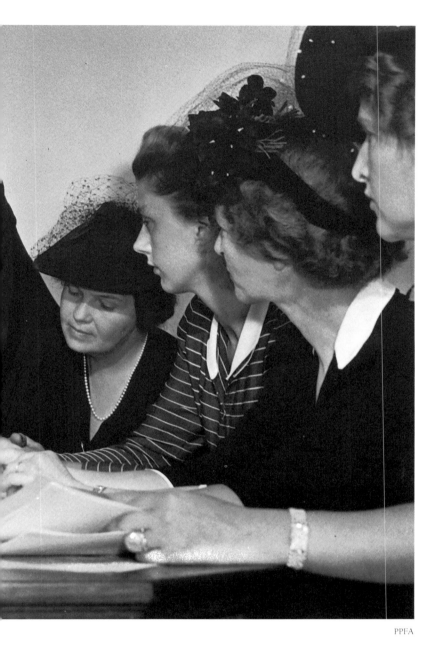

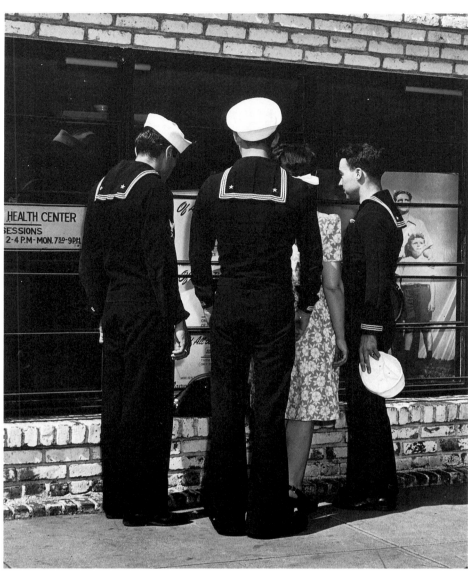

Young sailors and a young woman show interest in signs in the window of a Planned Parenthood affiliate in Jamaica, New York.

the war was over, insisting that it was women's duty to give up their jobs for men, go home and raise families. The Catholic church and other conservative religious groups exploited the argument for their own ends and effectively blocked any significant expansion of family planning services.

Adapting to the pronatalist climate, PPFA sought to convince the public that "Planned Parenthood" did not mean *smaller* families but, rather, *planned* families — and therefore healthier children. The April 1942 PPFA newsletter approvingly quoted a *Time*

magazine report on the impact of the state-sponsored family planning program in North Carolina:

"The purpose of North Carolina's birth control program has not been to cut down the state's birth rate — one of the highest in the country — but to increase the number of healthy newborn Tarheels. In five years, the State's stillbirths, maternal and infant death rates have dropped sharply. In counties where the birth control program reached a large number of women, the infant mortality rate dropped an average of 40 percent since 1937."

Always a strong supporter of women's rights, Eleanor Roosevelt was unafraid to express her pro-choice views even in the midst of controversy. The April 1945 Planned Parenthood News Exchange reprinted her detailed answer to charges that family planning would weaken America. She said: "Because the desire to have a family is a basic instinct, I believe we will always have enough babies to replenish our population if we can provide the right economic and social climate. That means making it possible for every mother to have a family of reasonable size, with some assurance that each child can be born well, can grow up healthy, receive a good education and have an opportunity to lead a useful and productive life....The emphasis of the Planned Parenthood movement, as far as I know, has never been on having fewer children but on planning for the birth of every child so that it will be born when the mother is well and strong enough and the family able to provide for it adequately."

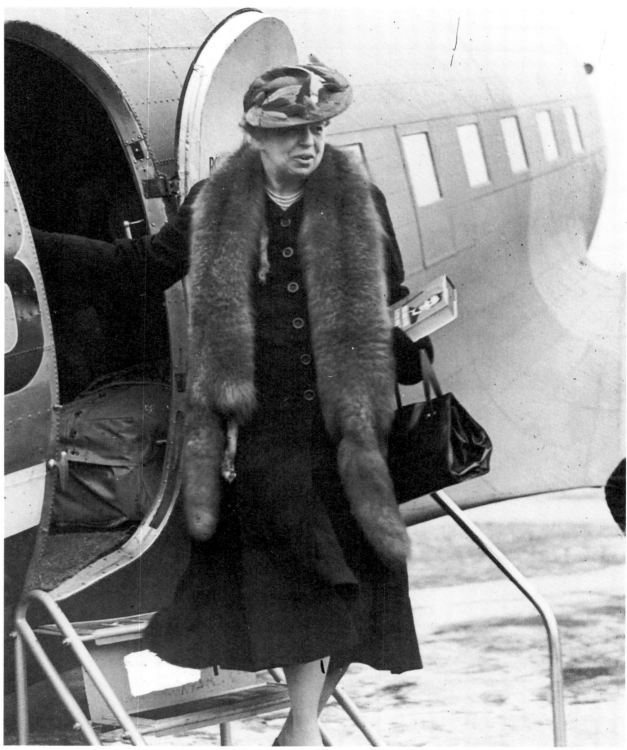

UPI/Bettmann

That North Carolina public health program was a model at a time when few state and county officials could be persuaded to accept, let alone finance, the provision of family planning services to poor women. Meanwhile, affiliates that raised private funds to provide services faced relentless harassment. Planned Parenthood of the St. Louis Region (Missouri) was a case in point.

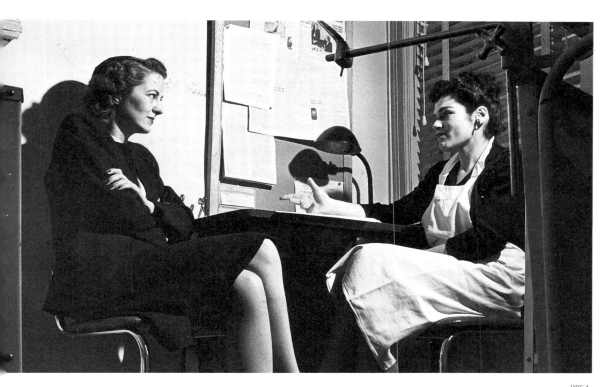

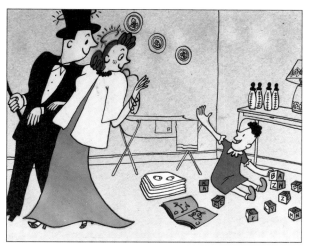

A slide from a 1946 film called "Happily Even After," produced by PPFA and emphasizing "the need for marriage counseling and family planning."

PPFA

This scene from a marriage counseling session at a Planned Parenthood affiliate appeared in a 1947 series on parenthood in **Look** magazine.

PPFA

Formed in 1932 as the Maternal Health Association by a group of devoted community leaders and professionals, by the mid-1940s, the affiliate had taken the name Planned Parenthood Association of Missouri and was operating four clinics, all in poor neighborhoods. In conformance with the city's Jim Crow laws and attitudes, the affiliate initially served black and white women in separate sessions. But in the postwar years, its board voted to change this policy and began to take a leadership role in the movement to integrate other public places in the city.

On April 22, 1945, Gladys Stockstrom, the organization's president, was confronted by an ad in the *St. Louis Dispatch*, paid for by the local Knights of Columbus, demanding that the Chamber of Commerce drop Planned Parenthood from its list of approved charities. Since Chamber of Commerce endorsement was an essential element in the affiliate's ability to provide services to indigent women, Stockstrom began to marshall community support for a hearing.

The case for reproductive choice was strengthened by a letter from an association of church and synagogue leaders that read in part:

"The local organization, as you doubtless know, complies with all the requirements of the Chamber in the management of its business....We feel quite strongly that the Chamber should not take sides in what is fundamentally a religious issue....The right of parents to use medically approved methods...should be a matter of individual conscience and decision. That is the democratic way."

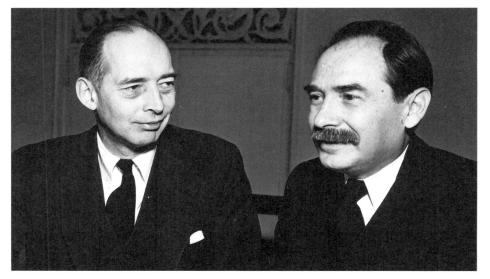

PPFA

Cornelius Trowbridge (left), chairperson of PPFA (1945-1948), and Abraham Stone, vice president of PPFA and director of the Birth Control Clinical Research Bureau, photographed at the 1947 annual meeting

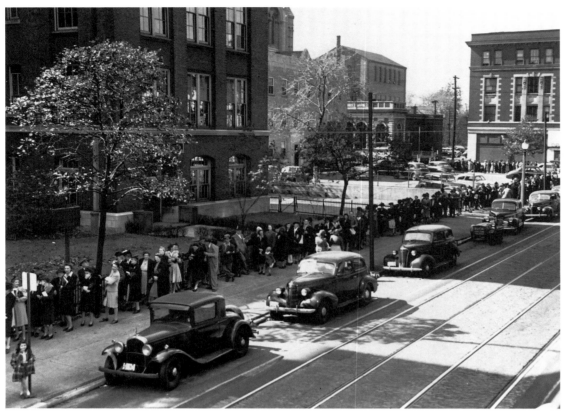

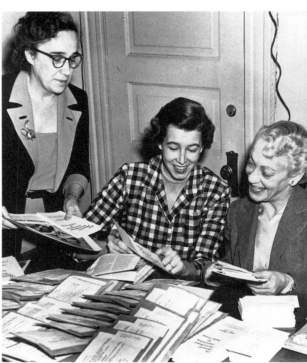

St. Louis residents stand on line for war rations in 1943. This photo was taken at 4458 Olive Street, a 10-minute drive from the first clinic operated by Planned Parenthood Association of Missouri (now Planned Parenthood of the St. Louis Region).

Staff and volunteers for Planned Parenthood Association of Missouri plan a fund-raising drive. The woman on the left is Mrs. Orville Sutter, whose spontaneous testimony on behalf of Planned Parenthood at a 1948 hearing stirred the crowd. Seated are Mrs. A. Wessel Shapleigh, Jr., and Mrs. Henry Stern.

July 23, 1948. A debate on whether Planned Parenthood should be allowed to continue operation in a public building in St. Louis packed this hearing room on a sweltering summer day.

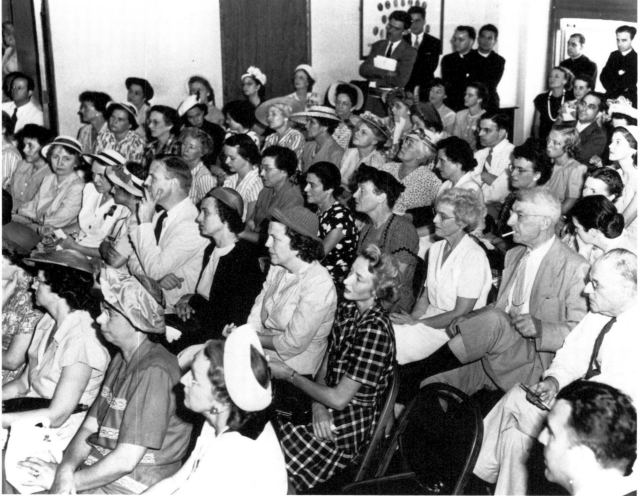

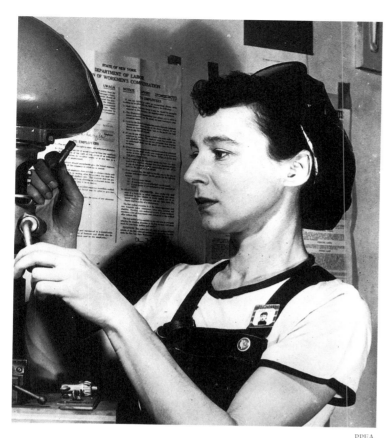

Elizabeth Hawes, a former fashion designer, working at a drill press in a defense plant during the war. Hawes's book, Why Women Cry — or Wenches with Wrenches, made a case for family planning services by stating, "One of the greatest fears of parents is that they may bring children into the world at the wrong time, when the mother is sick, the family unstable and unable to cope with another baby." She was a featured speaker at the 1944 PPFA annual meeting.

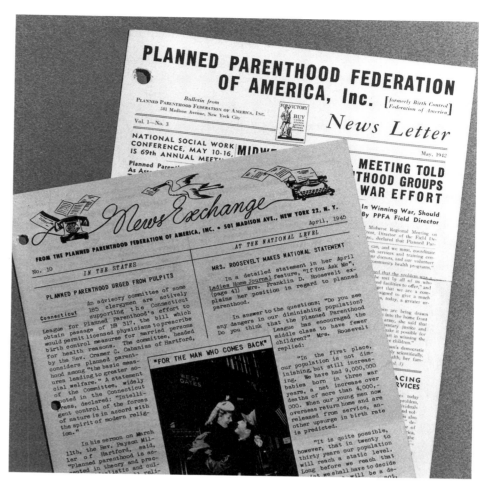

PPFA newsletters published during the war years (top) and immediately after the war (below)

The Chamber of Commerce ruled unanimously in favor of Planned Parenthood. But the troubles that St. Louis's poor women faced in obtaining family planning services continued. In spring 1949, antagonistic city officials actually managed to shut down a clinic for over a week. It reopened only after an intense letter-writing campaign and a threatened march on City Hall by clinic patients. Before reopening, the affiliate had to promise an outraged Catholic official that, in the future, only doctors and pharmacists — not volunteers — would hand a patient such a prescription item as a diaphragm!

In those difficult times, the outspoken support of ordinary citizens was a powerful force in sustaining the movement. Gladys Stockstrom recalled an occasion in 1948 when the county was attempting to oust a Planned Parenthood clinic from a public building and

her board was preparing for a hearing on that threat. A woman walked into the Planned Parenthood conference room and introduced herself as Mrs. Orville Sutter. She said, "My husband is a county employee and I am only a ten-dollar member but this is unfair. I will help in any way I can. I will speak this afternoon."

It was a sweltering afternoon in July, and the courthouse was packed, but Mrs. Sutter kept her word and attended the hearing. She rose and gave an eloquent speech, saying: "It is the right of every woman to limit her family, and Planned Parenthood gives women that opportunity."

While the clinic was not allowed back in the county building, it earned much favorable publicity from that hearing and gained enough support to resume operation in privately rented space.

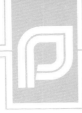

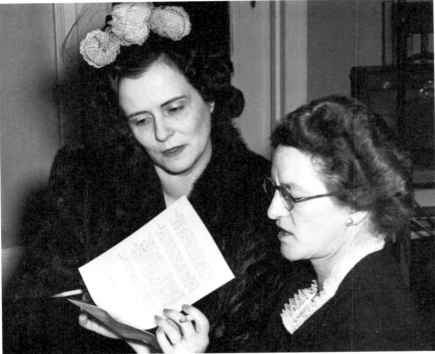

Mary (Mrs. Albert D.) Lasker (in hat) and Mrs. William Potter confer during fund-raising effort.

Tommy Weber/PPFA

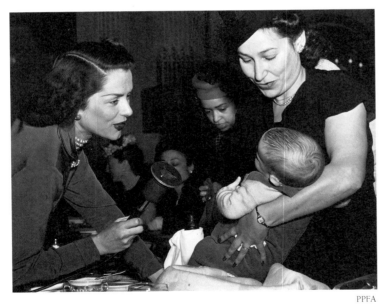

PPFA

Jinx Falkenburg (left), a well-known radio personality, interviews a Planned Parenthood volunteer on the theme of the 1948 fund-raising drive: "Planned Babies."

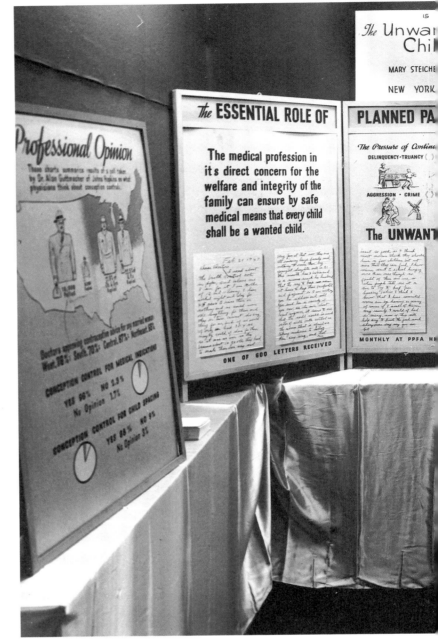

Display at a conference of the American College of Obstetricians and Gynecologists, held in St. Louis in 1947

Nationwide, the struggling affiliates of the 1940s were able to make only the slightest dent in the demand for birth control services. Thousands of men and women poured out their stories in letters to PPFA's main office, pleading for help in towns and rural areas where no help was to be had. One letter from a Nebraska woman read:

"Having read your item a year ago on birth control and being in desperate circumstances, I decided to come to you for help....

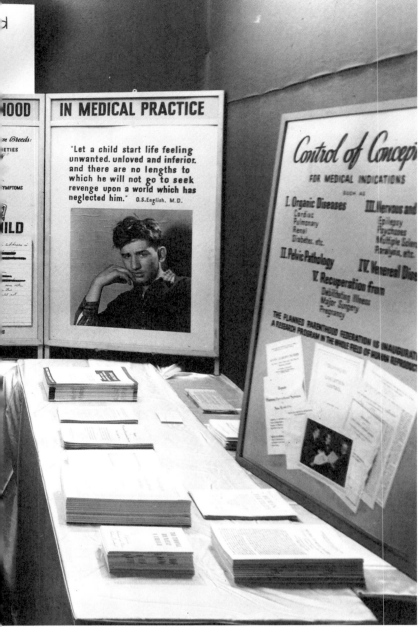

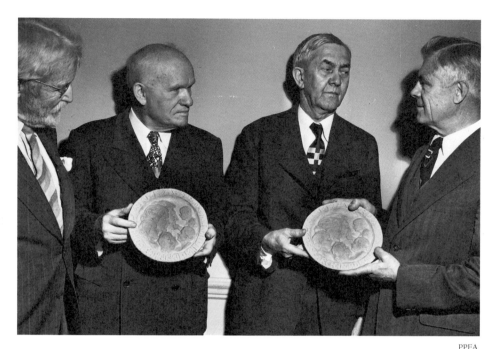

Charles E. Scribner (right), PPFA chairperson from 1948-1950, presenting the PPFA Lasker Award for conspicuous service to Dr. George W. Cooper of the North Carolina Health Department (second from right) and to researcher Dr. Carl G. Hartman. The medallions were the work of Dr. R. L. Dickinson (far left).

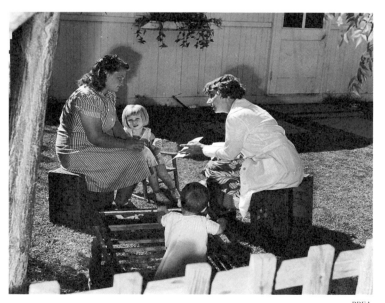

A Planned Parenthood field worker visits a woman in a rural area.

"The doctor told my husband I couldn't have any more [children] without losing my life, but wouldn't tell us anything to do. He said only an operation was safe....

"I can tell you my case is only one of the miseries that exist here in the West among us farm women and plenty in our towns....

"If there is such a place as a birth control clinic, I beg of you to tell me how and where I could get this information. If you would be kind enough to do me this favor and help me, I shall remember you every night in my prayers."

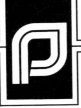

THE 1950s: "HUSH AND PRETEND"

"If the United States had spent two billion dollars developing...a contraceptive, instead of the atom bomb, it would have contributed far more to our national security while, at the same time, it promoted a rising living standard for the entire world. If such an amount is required to develop a satisfactory contraceptive, it will be a sound investment."

—William Vogt, PPFA national director 1950-1961

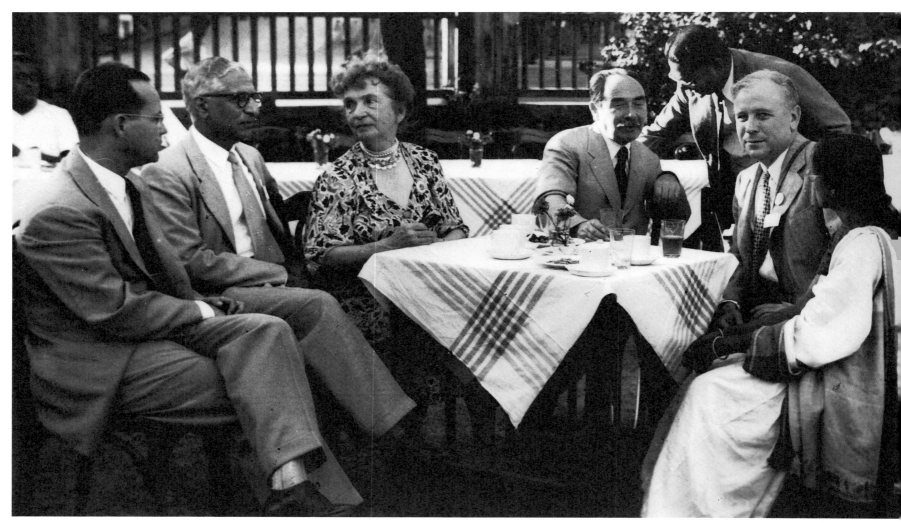

Margaret Sanger (third from left) and Abraham Stone (seated at Sanger's left) have lunch with international delegates during a break in the founding conference of the International Planned Parenthood Federation.

In the 1950s, conformity, complacency and the "feminine mystique" ruled America. Middle-class women were expected to be happy at home, with their up-to-the-minute electric dishwashers and cocktail shakers and the requisite three toddlers lapping up their boundless attention. Monroe shimmied and Presley gyrated — yet the age was a throwback to Victorian times, an era of "hush and pretend" (as historian James Reed put it), when sex was not discussed in polite company. No one suffered more from these attitudes than the nation's poor women, who, thanks to Planned Parenthood, by this time generally knew what a diaphragm was but were often hard-pressed to obtain one. Illegal abortion remained the only resort for many and the cause of countless injuries and deaths.

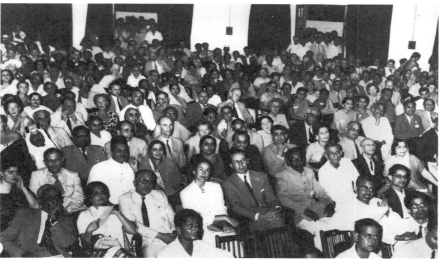

Delegates to the 1952 conference in Bombay, India, where the founding of IPPF was announced

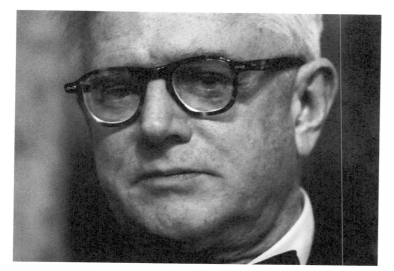

William Vogt (1902-1968)

Roy DeCarava/PPFA

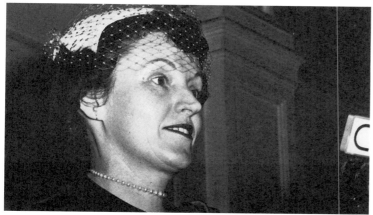

Jerry May/PPFA

Eleanor Pillsbury, PPFA chairperson from 1950-1954

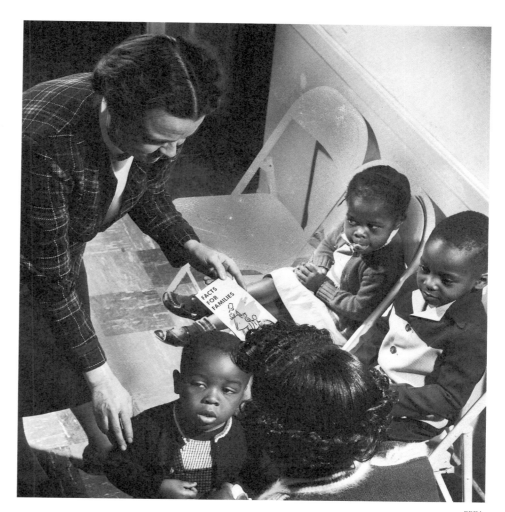

PPFA

A volunteer at the Denver clinic of Planned Parenthood of the Rocky Mountains cares for children while their mothers receive family planning services.

Meanwhile, on the international scene, scholars and leaders were waking up to the fact that the world's population was growing at an alarming rate and that women and families in developing countries urgently needed access to birth control. In 1952, concern over the impact of the world's population growth on human welfare and living standards, especially in developing countries, led to the founding of the Population Council. In the same year, the International Planned Parenthood Federation (IPPF), the first worldwide league of autonomous, indigenous family planning organizations, was founded at a conference in Bombay, India, with Margaret Sanger in a prominent role and PPFA as a founding member. But for many years, the United Nations and the U.S. government bowed to the pressure of religious groups by declining the pleas of foreign governments for family planning assistance.

In 1950, PPFA named as its new national director a man whose expertise on international population was widely recognized: William Vogt (1902-1968). Vogt, former chief of the conservation section of the Pan American Union, was best known as author of the 1948 best-seller, *Road to Survival*, one of the first popular works to bring ecological issues to the public's attention. A scholar and prolific writer, he had command over a range of subjects and statistics. Disabled by polio since the age of 14, he walked with a stick, twisting himself painfully from side to side. Pamela Veerhusen, executive director of Planned Parenthood of Minnesota in the middle 1950s, recalled, "He had enormous kindness and a keen sense of humor. You had the feeling that he had suffered and it made you listen to him."

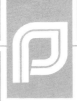

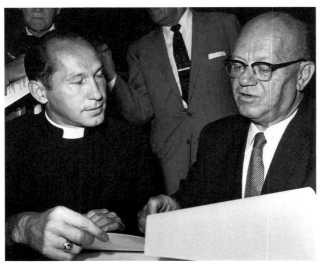

NYT Pictures

The New York City Public Hospitals Fight

The Rev. Dan Potter, executive director of the New York City Protestant Council, presents petitions to Morris Jacobs, New York City commissioner of hospitals, requesting that New York City public hospitals begin providing birth control services to indigent women who seek that help.

The petition drive was part of a fight that began in December 1956, when Dr. Louis Hellman (1908-1990), chief obstetrician at Kings County Hospital in Brooklyn, asked his hospital, the largest in the city's public system, to start a contraceptive service. Hellman's board approved the request. But when Commissioner Jacobs, fearing the wrath of the Catholic church, hedged, PPFA organized a coalition of media representatives and religious, medical and community groups to support Hellman.

With the quiet backing of this community coalition and the eager cooperation of the media, Hellman announced that on July 16, 1958, he would fit a diaphragm on a diabetic mother of three whose life would be threatened by another pregnancy. No objection was raised to his announcement — but on that day as he was about to proceed, he received a telephone call with the news that the commissioner had forbidden him to go ahead.

A media controversy raged through the summer of 1958. As public awareness grew that the Catholic church had for years been inflicting a cruel and dogmatic policy on the thousands of women dependent on the public health system — most of whom were not even Catholic — the city began to soften its position. Finally, in September 1958, the hospital commission voted 8-2 to reverse its ban. While it remained very difficult for poor women in most major metropolitan areas to get access to services, this highly publicized victory in the nation's media capital raised hopes across the country.

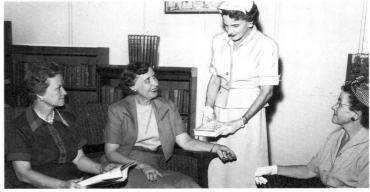

PPFA

A biography of Margaret Sanger by Lawrence Lader, published by Doubleday in 1955, catalyzed an outreach initiative by Planned Parenthood affiliates, who gave away many copies to schools and libraries. In this publicity photo, volunteer leaders of the Planned Parenthood Center of San Angelo, Texas (standing and seated, far left), present the book to local librarians.

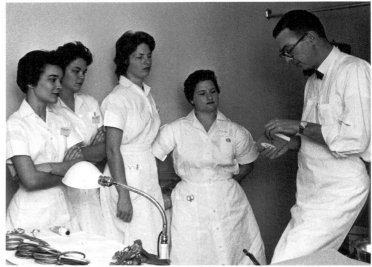

Bert Brandt V Associates/PPFA

In this 1955 photo taken at the clinic of Planned Parenthood of Houston and Southeastern Texas, Dr. Harold Secor explains contraceptive techniques to nursing students. The Houston affiliate today operates 16 clinics serving nearly 30,000 clients annually.

To combat the repressive attitudes of the day and raise the movement's visibility, Vogt launched an aggressive public affairs program. This included an array of new publications on sexuality education, cooperative efforts with many national and community organizations and a strong media campaign to put Planned Parenthood's mission and services before the public. Key figures in developing these new initiatives were two vice presidents who became known to the New York media as "the birth control boys": Frederick S. Jaffe (1925-1978) and Winfield Best.

Meanwhile, affiliates won acceptability by

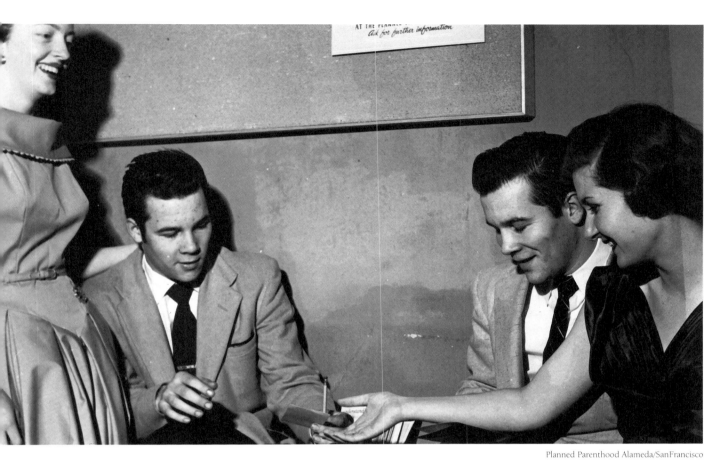

Engaged and newly married couples talk about planning children at a session called "Understanding Marriage" at Planned Parenthood Alameda/San Francisco. Just a decade later, with the counterculture in full bloom around it, this affiliate would become the first in the nation to establish a clinic especially to meet the needs of teenagers for sexuality information and family planning services.

Planned Parenthood Alameda/SanFrancisco

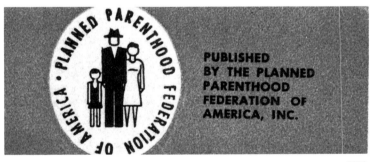

PPFA

The PPFA logo in the early 1950s. Note the placement of the man squarely at the center of the family, reflecting the attitudes of the day about male leadership.

featuring less controversial services, such as marriage counseling and infertility treatment. They managed to survive and grow, with an annual patient load that swelled from 46,000 in 1949 to 117,000 in 1959. Despite the careful emphasis on keeping husbands happy and babies healthy, 80 percent of all patients came for contraceptive services — which in those days meant the diaphragm and jelly, condoms or contraceptive foam. Though some affiliates quietly served single and divorced women, most Planned Parenthood patients described themselves as married, and the majority already had children.

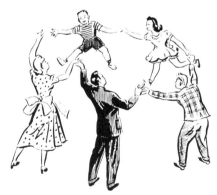

You are invited to
ATTEND OUR CHILD SPACING CLINIC
OR SECURE A LIST OF SPECIALISTS

"The happy family—we planned it that way."

Call MAin 4480
Monday through Friday, 9 to 5 o'clock

PLANNED PARENTHOOD CENTER
311 Lyon Building, Third at James Street

"CHILDREN BY CHOICE RATHER THAN BY CHANCE"

PPFA

A flyer distributed by Planned Parenthood of Seattle-King County in the 1950s

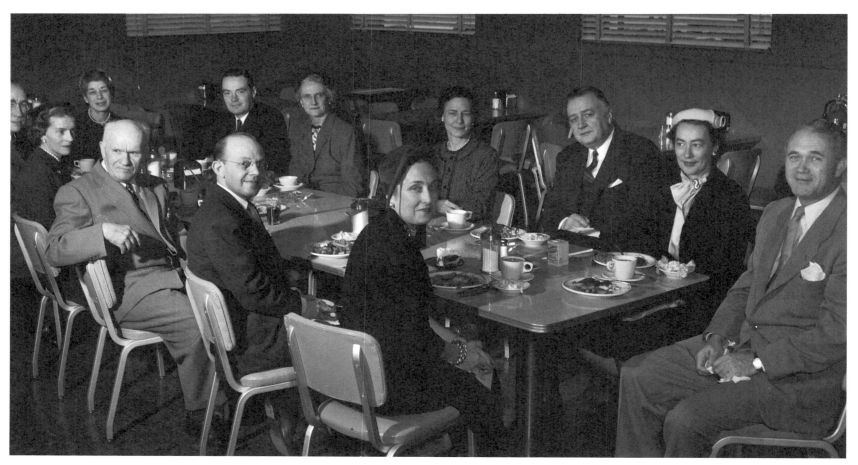

PPFA board members discussed contraceptive research with Ortho Research Foundation staff during a 1956 visit to the Ortho Research Foundation in Raritan, New Jersey. Ortho at the time had a million-dollar medical research program of which one-fifth was devoted to the development and testing of contraceptives.

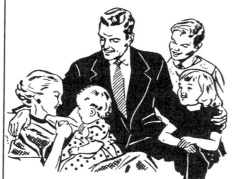

helping you to have your children
when it's best for **you** *and* **them!**

PLANNED PARENTHOOD CLINIC

OF PITTSBURGH

108 SMITHFIELD STREET

Phone **ATlantic 1-9502**

a non-profit health service organization

This car card was displayed on 299 street cars in Pittsburgh in 1954 — marking a breakthrough in public acceptance of Planned Parenthood advertising.

Because family planning services remained inaccessible to most women who needed them, Planned Parenthood affiliates employed staff and volunteers as field workers. They canvassed homes in rural areas and poor urban communities and set up movable clinics in a variety of community settings. For example, in 1955, in a pioneering project in New Jersey's potato belt, the New Jersey League for Planned Parenthood obtained the cooperation of a minister to offer weekly contraceptive services for migrant farm workers in a church.

Eloise Whitten, a longtime Planned Parenthood board member and activist, recalled organizing "Planned Parenthood tea parties" in housing projects in Detroit, Michigan, where she would explain to tenants the safest and most effective methods of birth control and how to obtain them. She said:

"I didn't feel I was joining anything controversial. Women in my family and

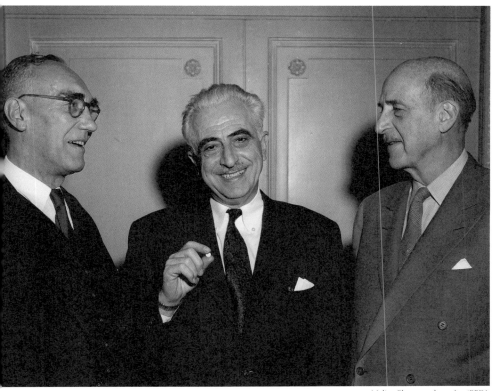

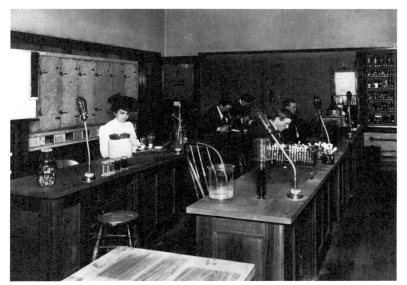

Katharine Dexter McCormick, whose passionate interest and financial support made possible the development of the first oral contraceptive, is shown here in a photo from the early 1900s, as the only young woman in the chemistry lab of Massachusetts Institute of Technology.

Dr. Gregory Pincus, one of the scientists involved in development of the first oral contraceptive, holds a birth control pill before the camera as General William Draper and Cass Canfield, PPFA board chairperson (1959-1962), look on.

neighborhood had died from not having birth control. The real problem was that people didn't know that Planned Parenthood existed.

"The ladies I talked to didn't know much about birth control. They thought you could lose a diaphragm inside your body. At that time, the social services office would close a case if a woman got pregnant, because they considered that evidence that she was providing an unsuitable environment for her children. But they wouldn't help her to get birth control."

Unfortunately, efforts to extend reproductive choice to women in America and internationally were blocked by more than opposition and ignorance — they were hindered just as much by the limitations of the available methods of contraception. Women in the 1950s were still using the methods of the 1920s, and the compelling need for more and better birth control options was clear to virtually everyone who cared about women's reproductive health and rights. In the 1940s and 1950s, Margaret Sanger closely followed scientific research on birth control and personally funded some of it, while PPFA made support for new birth control technology a major focus of its advocacy efforts. The turning point came, though, when a remarkable woman named Katharine Dexter McCormick (1875-1967) threw her support behind research to produce an oral contraceptive.

McCormick, heir to the International Harvester fortune, was one of the first women graduates of the Massachusetts Institute of Technology, an ardent supporter of women's rights and a longtime friend of Sanger. In 1950, following the death of her husband, Stanley, McCormick wrote to Sanger to ask how she could use her inheritance to contribute to contraceptive research.

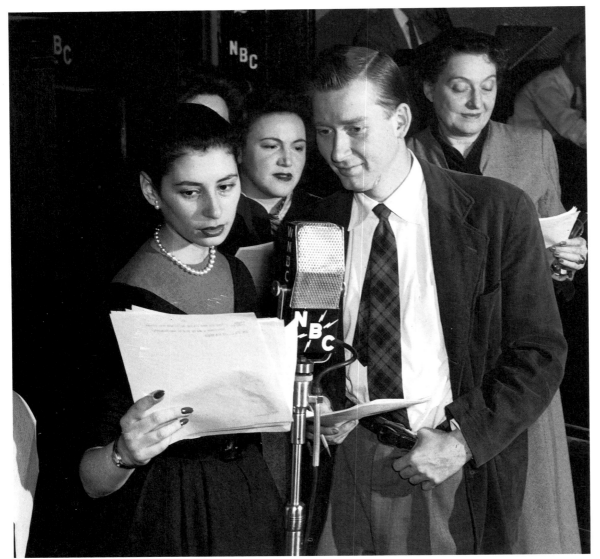

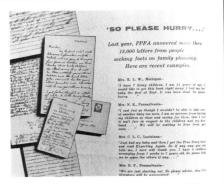

PPFA

Just as the American Birth Control League was the place to which desperate women wrote for help in the 1920s, PPFA was the recipient of thousands of poignant letters in later years. A few examples, reprinted in the 1957 newsletter where this graphic appeared, read:

"I have 7 living children. I am 31 years of age and would like to get this [birth control information] right away. I had my last baby the first of Sept. It was born dead. So please hurry."

"I just feel as though I wouldn't be able to take care of another baby too soon. I am so nervous from having my children so close and caring for them, that I feel it isn't fair in respect to the children and my husband."

"I halve 3 children now and expectin my fourth in 6 years time. I wood lack to find out about putting a fue more years between my children. I love children but I halvin them to fast."

Rosen Studios/PPFA

Professional actors record a 15-minute radio script, "Happiness Is a Way of Life," a 1955 promotional piece that told the story of a young couple whose marriage was saved by visiting a Planned Parenthood clinic.

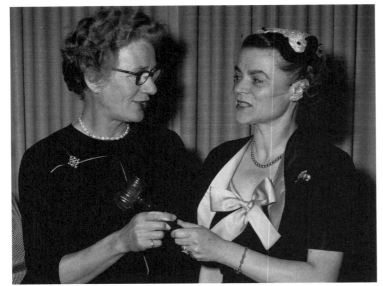

Meljay Photographers/PPFA

At the 1956 annual meeting, Loraine Campbell (left), newly elected chairperson of PPFA, accepts the gavel from Frances Ferguson, outgoing chairperson.

In 1953, Sanger took McCormick to visit the Worcester Foundation in Massachusetts, where research scientists Gregory Pincus and Min Chueh Chang were conducting experiments Sanger considered promising, attempting to produce an oral contraceptive based on synthetic progesterone. McCormick first pledged them $10,000. Soon after, she began contributing $150,000 to $180,000 a year, funneling a portion of the money through PPFA's research grant program.

McCormick also funded the first clinical trials of the pill, which were conducted by Dr. John Rock, an eminent Catholic gynecologist, with patients in his private practice. Rock, who came to be regarded as a co-developer of

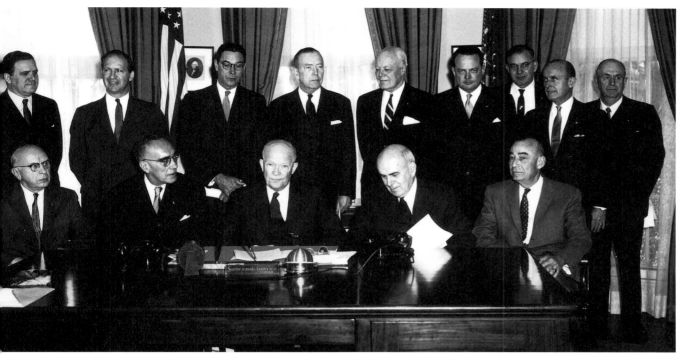

The 1959 Draper commission on foreign aid was appointed by President Dwight D. Eisenhower (seated at center) and headed by General William Draper (at Eisenhower's right). The commission recommended that family planning aid should be made available to foreign governments that requested it as part of development aid. President Eisenhower rejected this proposal, saying, "I cannot imagine anything more emphatically a subject that is not a proper political or governmental activity or function or responsibility."

Draper, however, went on to become a leading advocate of family planning aid for developing countries and ultimately converted Eisenhower to his point of view. To raise funds and support for international population efforts, Draper co-founded the World Population Emergency Campaign (WPEC), which merged with PPFA in 1962. In 1964, Eisenhower publicly retracted his 1959 statement and agreed to serve as co-chair of the honorary sponsors' council of PPFA-WPEC, together with the only other then-living ex-president, Harry S. Truman.

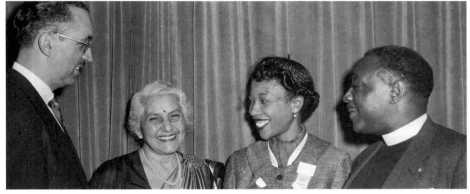

Scene from the 1955 PPFA annual meeting. Lady Rama Rau (second from left) was the leading figure in India's family planning movement and the first president of IPPF. Naomi Gray (second from right) was at the time a PPFA field consultant; she later became vice president. Flanking the two women are William Trent (left), executive director of the United Negro College Fund, and the Rev. James H. Robinson (right), Church of the Master, New York.

the pill, worked with PPFA staff on a closely reasoned book, *The Time Has Come,* arguing that the Catholic church should accept the oral contraceptive as a natural extension of the rhythm method.

In 1956, the journal *Science* announced the success of Rock's clinical trials. Four years later, the Food and Drug Administration (FDA) approved distribution of the Enovid contraceptive pill, manufactured by G.D. Searle and Company, a firm that had also supported Gregory Pincus's research for many years.

The birth control pill was far from perfect — but its effectiveness, simplicity and ease of use extended to millions of women an

unheard-of control over reproduction, for the first time allowing them to truly separate the sexual act from procreation. As Sanger wrote McCormick in 1956, after the success of Rock's clinical trials was announced in *Science*:

"You must, indeed, feel a certain pride in your judgment. Gregory Pincus had practically no money for this work and Dr. [Abraham] Stone and I did our best to get a few dollars for him. Then you came along with your fine interest and enthusiasm and your faith and things began to happen and at last the reports are now out in the outstanding scientific magazine. The conspiracy of silence has been broken."

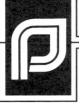

THE 1960s: THE BREAKTHROUGH YEARS

"We have passed a historic turning point in thinking about programs concerned with Planned Parenthood and population growth....The responsibility of the federal government in the area of family planning and world population problems has been clearly stated by the President on at least 20 occasions."

—Wilbur J. Cohen, undersecretary, Department of Health, Education and Welfare in the Lyndon Johnson administration

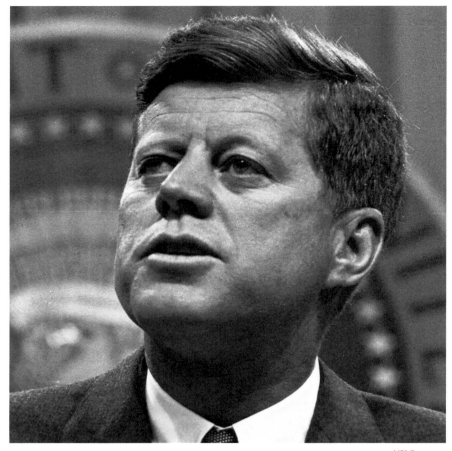

UPI/Bettmann

John F. Kennedy (1917-1963) was the first sitting U.S. president to formally endorse birth control technology. He called for expanded research into human reproduction that would make knowledge "available to the world so everyone can make his own decision."

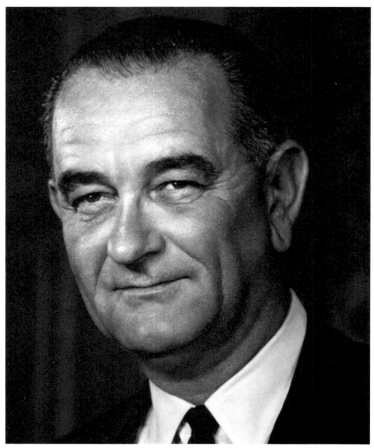

The Bettmann Archive

As president, Lyndon B. Johnson (1908-1973) was a staunch advocate of expanding access to family planning services and population assistance. The first federal grants for services in the U.S. and in developing countries came during his administration and with his support.

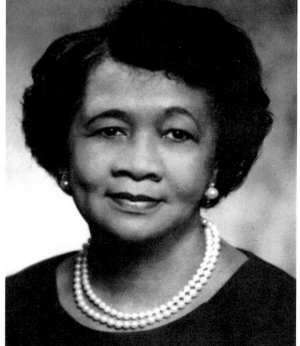

National Council of Negro Women

Dorothy Height, president of the National Council of Negro Women, served as a member of PPFA's national board in the 1960s.

In the 1960s, the impassioned demands of African-Americans for social justice awakened the American conscience. The Vietnam War gave rise to massive protests. A new youth "counterculture" rebelled against the mores of an older generation and women began to protest the subservient roles handed down to them from the postwar generation. A refreshing new frankness about sexuality, growing concern over worldwide population growth and a revolution in contraceptive technology all contributed to a sea change in national attitudes toward family planning and, by the decade's end, a substantial expansion of the tradition of choice.

The feeling of fresh air that characterized the family planning movement in the 1960s was visibly symbolized by the dynamic new leader selected by the PPFA national board in 1962. Alan F. Guttmacher, M.D. (1898-1974),

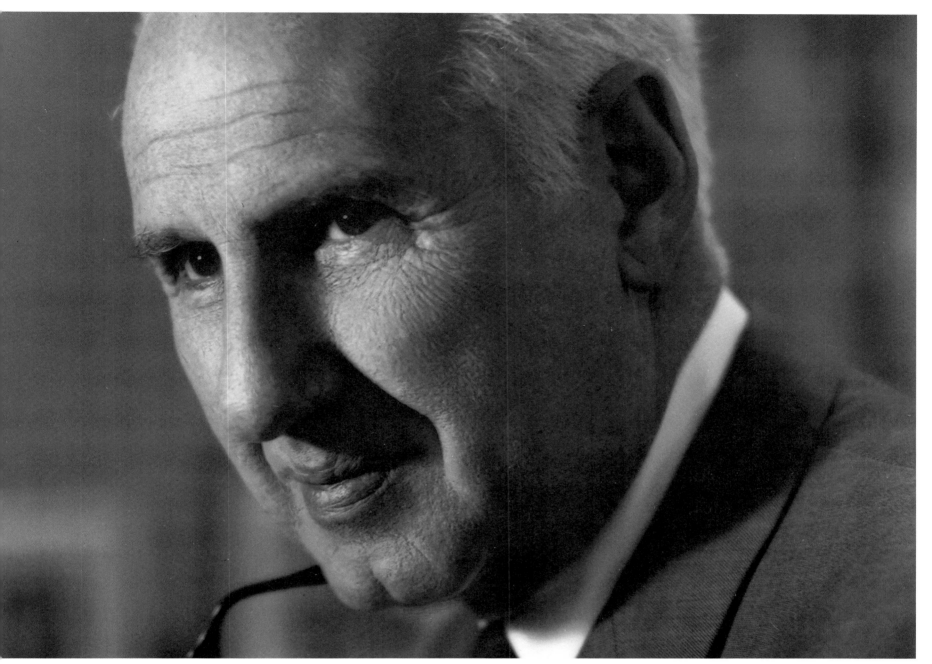

Alan Guttmacher (1898-1974)

was a distinguished gynecologist and well-known writer on the subject of sex and marriage, whose outspoken advocacy of birth control dated back to the 1930s. The son of a rabbi and a social worker, Guttmacher addressed his subject with infectious enthusiasm, formidable knowledge and an engaging, down-to-earth style that captivated both the media and grass-roots supporters.

As a medical researcher, Guttmacher was an early champion of the intrauterine device (IUD), which was introduced to patients in the U.S. and developing countries early in the 1960s. Along with the oral contraceptive, this convenient new form of birth control, which could remain in place in the uterus for several years after insertion by a practitioner, prompted an upsurge in the popularity of Planned Parenthood and family planning. By the end of the decade, the number of Planned Parenthood contraceptive patients had nearly tripled, to more than 345,000, and 90 percent of all contraceptive patients were choosing either the pill or the IUD.

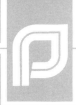

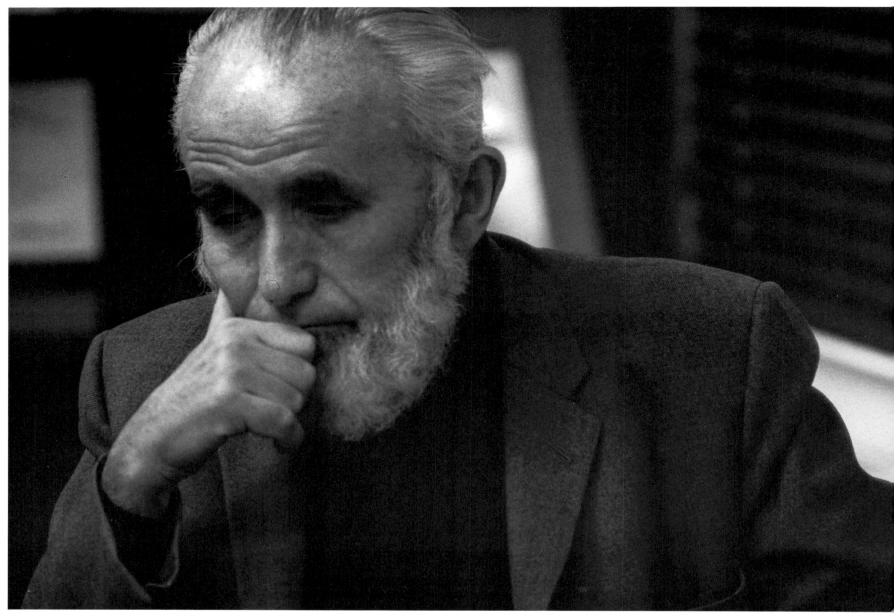

Edwin Snyder/PPFA

Christopher Tietze (1908-1984), a brilliant medical statistician initially associated with the Johns Hopkins School of Public Health and later with the Population Council and other family planning organizations, devoted most of his life to studying methods of improving reproductive health. His research and publications helped lead to approval of the intrauterine device (IUD) and to widespread recognition of the health benefits of legal abortion.

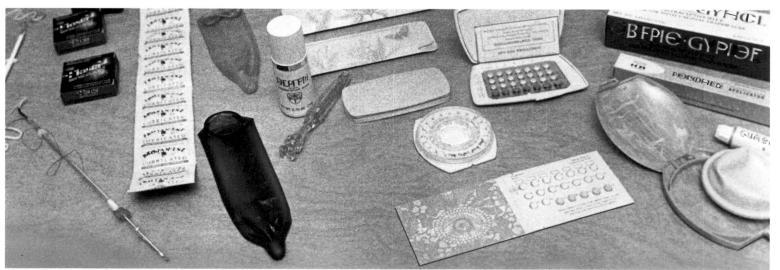

Birth control methods available at the end of the 1960s

PPFA

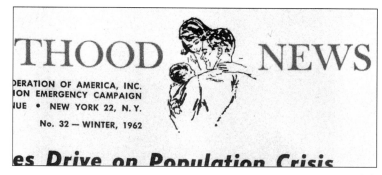

PPFA

In 1959, Planned Parenthood adopted a new logo, which still showed a strong male presence but no longer had a man towering over a woman.

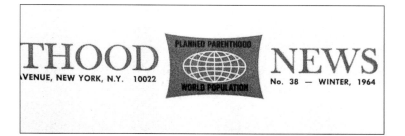

PPFA

After PPFA merged with the World Population Emergency Campaign, an organization founded by General William Draper to support international family planning efforts, it began using the name "Planned Parenthood–World Population" on its newsletter and annual reports, along with a new logo of a bulging globe.

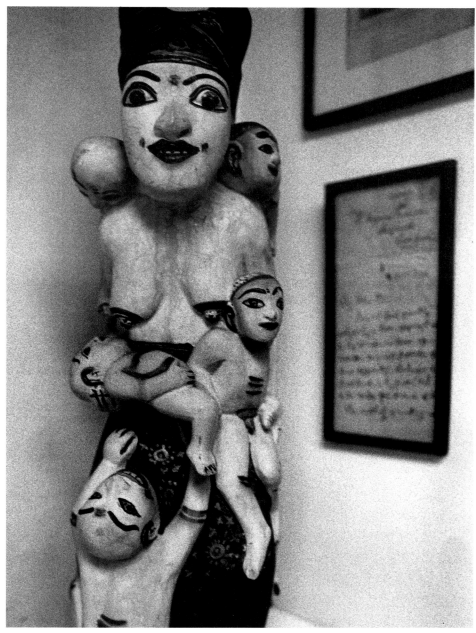

Tim Kantor/PPFA

An Indonesian fertility goddess that Alan Guttmacher kept on display in his office at PPFA

Breakthroughs in public policy succeeded each other in rapid order, many of them driven by new awareness of the phenomenon of rapid population growth and the danger it posed to the planet's future. A turning point in the U.S. Congress took place in 1963, when the first vote in favor of family planning was recorded, in the form of majority support for an amendment to the foreign aid bill to permit the use of funds for population research. Then, in 1964, the Office of Economic Opportunity, established by Congress to conduct the War on Poverty, granted the first funds ever to support domestic family planning programs. The next year, when the Medicaid program passed Congress, it also permitted states to treat family planning as a reimbursable service.

Guttmacher capitalized on the favorable Washington, D.C., climate by establishing the first Washington office of PPFA, under the direction of Frederick S. Jaffe and with Jeannie I. Rosoff as the first lobbyist. This office soon became an autonomous institute, the Center for Family Planning Program Development — and eventually, after Guttmacher's death in 1974, The Alan Guttmacher Institute (AGI). Its solid, scholarly research uncovered sobering facts. In the middle 1960s, Jaffe and Rosoff found that across the nation, 4.5 million sexually active American women who needed and wanted to avoid pregnancy had no access to family planning services, because they could not afford private care and no affordable source of services was close enough.

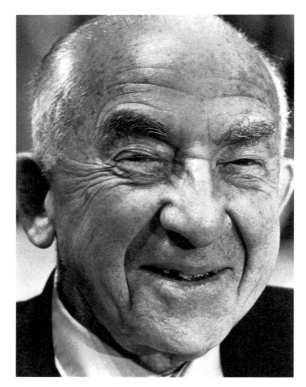

UPI/Bettmann

Senator Ernest F. Gruening of Alaska (1887-1974) was also a medical doctor, whose commitment to the birth control movement dated to his student days at Harvard Medical School in the early 1900s. From 1965-1968, he held a series of Senate subcommittee hearings on population that focused public attention on family planning issues and helped pave the way for passage of Title X.

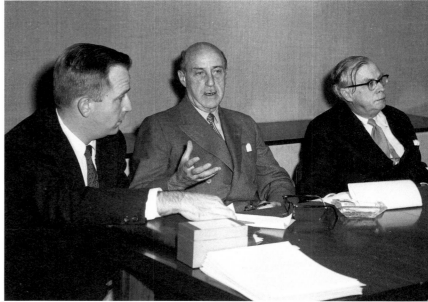

Meljay Photographers, Inc./PPFA

Frederick Jaffe (left), the PPFA vice president who was the first president of The Alan Guttmacher Institute, with Cass Canfield (center), PPFA chairperson, and Julian Huxley, the famed British biologist and writer

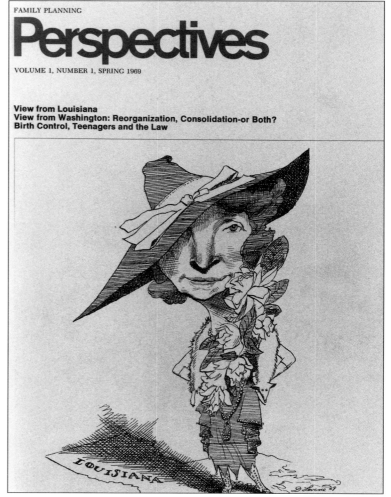

FAMILY PLANNING

Perspectives

VOLUME 1, NUMBER 1, SPRING 1969

View from Louisiana
View from Washington: Reorganization, Consolidation-or Both?
Birth Control, Teenagers and the Law

The Alan Guttmacher Institute

Family Planning Perspectives, the essential scholarly journal in the field of family planning and population, was first published in spring 1969 by The Alan Guttmacher Institute (AGI). Known then as the Center for Family Planning Program Development, AGI today is an independent, nonprofit corporation for research, policy analysis and public education on reproductive health issues and a special affiliate of PPFA.

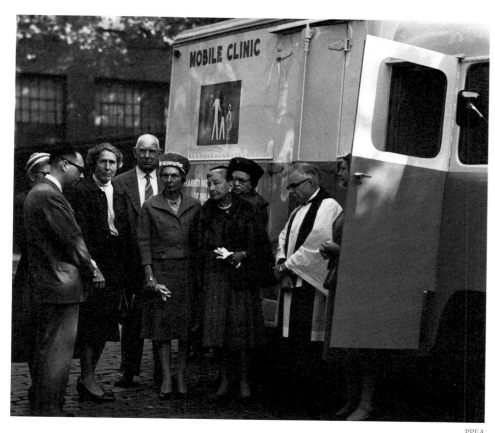

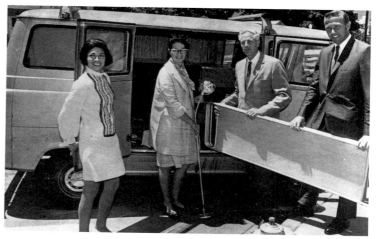

Planned Parenthood Assoc. of San Mateo County

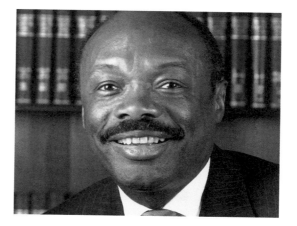

At a time when family planning services were inaccessible to millions of the nation's poor, Planned Parenthood affiliates helped fill the gap by pioneering mobile units, equipped with all the necessities for setting up a temporary family planning clinic in a church, a community center or any other place that had electricity and running water. Shown here are the mobile units of Planned Parenthood of Southeastern Pennsylvania (Philadelphia), above, and San Mateo County (California), above right. Another pioneer in the use of these vans was Planned Parenthood of Chicago, which in 1962 set up clinics at four settlement houses and a community health council.

PPFA

Willie L. Brown, Jr., speaker of the California State Assembly, served as a member of PPFA's national board from 1968-1974.

PPFA made this finding the basis of a vigorous campaign, calling for a far wider *choice* of services for people at all levels of income — not just through Planned Parenthood affiliates, but at public and private hospitals, clinics, social welfare offices and virtually every other site where people came for health care or service referrals. Only in this way, when access to family planning became truly universal, would American women at all levels of income finally achieve the freedom from unwanted childbearing that affluent and many middle-class women had. By the end of the decade, this bold vision was nearing realization: Title X of the Public Health Service Act was about to be passed with overwhelming bipartisan support.

Meanwhile, a case against an old Comstock law brought by the Planned Parenthood League of Connecticut (PPLC), now called Planned Parenthood of Connecticut, Inc., was wending its way to the U.S. Supreme Court. Called *Griswold v. Connecticut*, it arose from the startling fact that — although contraceptive methods were by this time readily prescribed and sold in most states — Connecticut's 1879 Comstock statute still prevented women in that state from obtaining or using birth control. The Connecticut State Legislature had repeatedly refused to change the law, and the highest court in Connecticut had upheld it, on the grounds that women had a "workable alternative" to contraception — abstention from sex. As a result, the only way PPLC could provide services legally was to escort women over the state border to clinics in Rhode Island and New York.

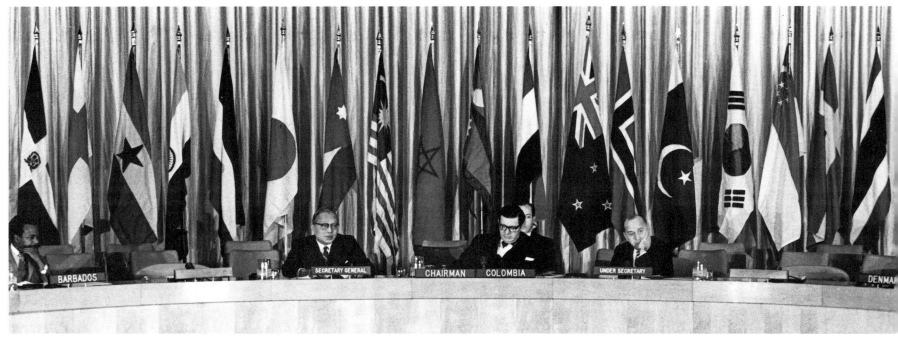

United Nations

The World Leaders' Declaration on Population, signed by the heads of state or prime ministers of 30 nations, is presented to the United Nations on December 11, 1967.

In 1966, the year of Margaret Sanger's death at the age of 87, the PPFA Margaret Sanger Award was established. Planned Parenthood's highest honor, the award recognizes excellence and leadership in the fields of reproductive health and reproductive rights. The actual award, shown here, is a bronze statuette called Children of the World by the artist Stanley Bleifeld.

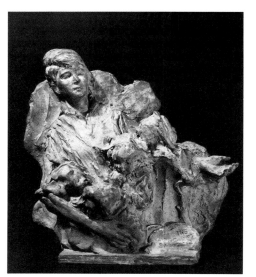

Soichi Sunami/PPFA

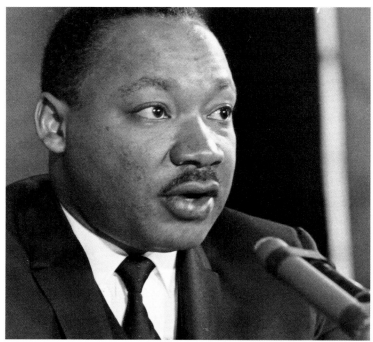

AP/World Wide Photos

A recipient of the PPFA Margaret Sanger Award in the year it was established, Martin Luther King, Jr., acknowledged the tribute with these words: "There is scarcely anything more tragic in human life than a child who is not wanted. That which should be a blessing becomes a curse for parent and child. Negroes have a special and urgent concern with family planning as a profoundly important ingredient in their struggle for security and a decent life. Our sure beginning in the struggle for equality by nonviolent action may not have been so resolute without the tradition established by Mrs. Sanger."

In 1961, Estelle Griswold, executive director of PPLC, convinced her board of directors to support a direct challenge to the law. On November 1, she and Dr. Charles Lee Buxton, chairman of the Yale School of Medicine Department of Obstetrics and Gynecology, opened a birth control clinic in New Haven. Like Margaret Sanger in Brownsville, they served crowds of eager women before being arrested by the police.

The landmark case that resulted was decided by the Supreme Court in 1965. Justice William O. Douglas wrote the majority opinion:

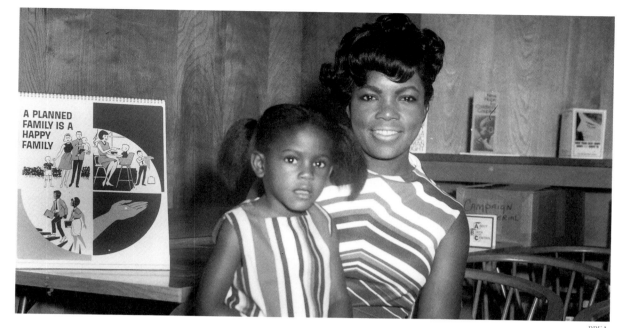

In the 1960s, Planned Parenthood clients included Mrs. John D. Batie of Houston, Texas, shown here with her child, and quoted in the PPFA newsletter as saying, "My husband is in school now and if it were not for Planned Parenthood, this would not be possible. We have one child now and are planning to have more." Among the patients who wrote to thank Planned Parenthood in the 1960s were: a 31-year-old field hand from Phoenix who had 11 children and worked at her husband's side on lettuce and cotton crops, even while pregnant; a 30-year-old Detroit woman whose husband was unemployed and who had seen four of her 11 children die; and a 30-year old Rhode Island woman with four children who credited Planned Parenthood with saving her marriage by relieving the fear of another unwanted pregnancy.

PPFA

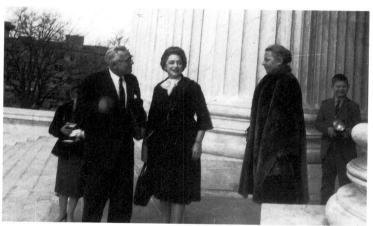

Collection of Mary H. Dodge

Harriet Pilpel, who represented PPFA in the case of Griswold v. Connecticut (1965), pauses on the steps of the U.S. Supreme Court between Lee Buxton and Estelle Griswold, who in 1961 were charged with operating a birth control clinic in New Haven in violation of Connecticut's Comstock law. Thomas Emerson argued the case for the Planned Parenthood League of Connecticut; Fowler Harper and Catherine Roraback did much of the legal work in preparation for the case.

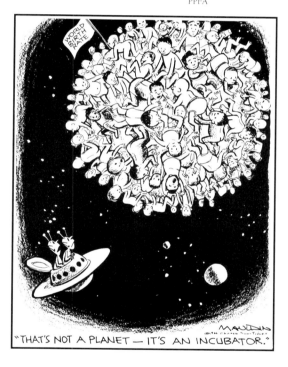

"THAT'S NOT A PLANET — IT'S AN INCUBATOR."

The prospect of rapid population growth, as it appeared to a cartoonist in 1966

Reprinted with permission from *Chicago Sun Times*

"We deal with a right of privacy older than the Bill of Rights — older than our political parties, older than our school system. Marriage is a coming together, for better or for worse, hopefully enduring and intimate to the degree of being sacred."

The state, Douglas concluded, was constitutionally barred from interfering with a married couple's decision about childbearing.

The decision in *Griswold* at last enabled married women in Connecticut to get contraceptive services. (Unmarried people were not granted the same right until the Supreme Court's 1972 decision in *Eisenstadt v. Baird*.) But the ruling accomplished an even larger purpose. By identifying a constitutional right of privacy that no state could violate, *Griswold* barred family planning opponents from imposing legal restrictions on access to services in the future. And *Griswold* did one more thing: it laid the ground for affirming the right to safe and legal abortion, opening the gates to the next major chapter in the tradition of choice.

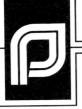

THE 1970s: SAFE AND LEGAL AT LAST

"I will never forget a patient who came to us for birth control pills in the 1960s — a young black woman with three children, all under the age of three. They were living in a single-room flat where the baby slept in a dresser drawer. She did diapers for the three children in a sink in the corner of the room. But her husband had a training position and two jobs and things were looking up for them. She was so excited about the possibility of a new life. Then we gave her a pelvic exam and discovered that she was pregnant again. And that woman just fell apart in my arms. She was absolutely desolate and there wasn't anything I could do. Abortion was illegal, unless a woman could afford a trip to Japan, which cost about $1,000, and she didn't have 10 cents."

—Lee Minto, president, Planned Parenthood Seattle-King County

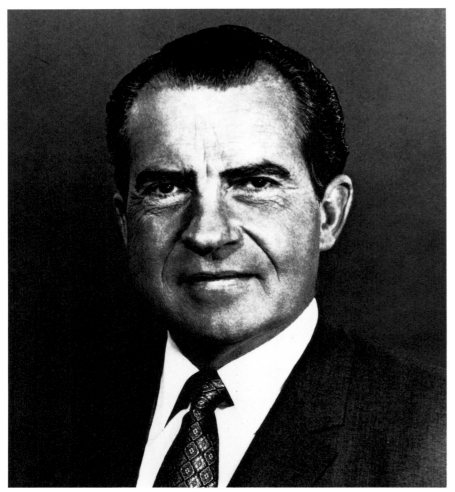

UPI/Bettmann

At the end of 1970, President Richard M. Nixon signed into law Title X of the Public Health Service Act, which was designed to provide universal access to family planning services.

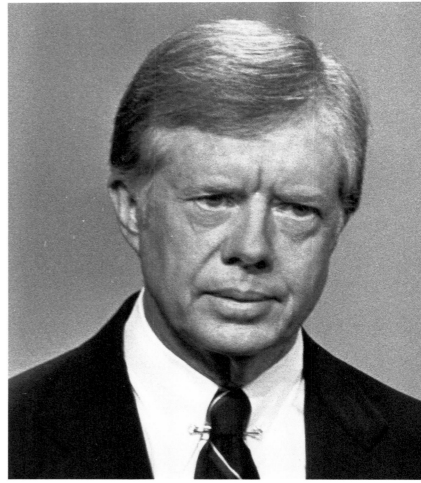

UPI/Bettmann Newsphotos

During the administration of President Jimmy Carter, the mandate of Title X was expanded to include services to teens.

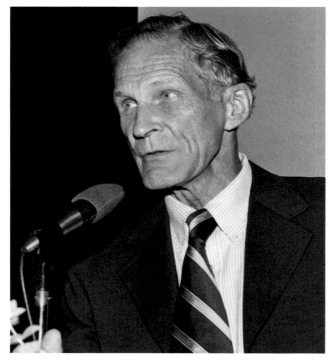

Edward H. Goldberger/PPFA

Alan Sweezey, PPFA chairperson from 1972-1975

It was the decade when major civil rights and equal opportunity legislation was passed, when the U.S. military finally withdrew from Vietnam, when the Watergate scandal caused the downfall of one U.S. president and the seizure of hostages in Iran led to the downfall of another. It was a momentous time as well for the reproductive rights movement.

On Christmas Eve 1970, President Richard Nixon signed into law the first federal legislation specifically designed to expand access to family planning services: Title X of the Public Health Service Act. The bill had been sponsored in Congress by then-Representative George Bush (Republican-Texas), Representative James Scheuer (Democrat-New York) and Senator Joseph Tydings (Democrat-Maryland), leading President Nixon to note that "this landmark

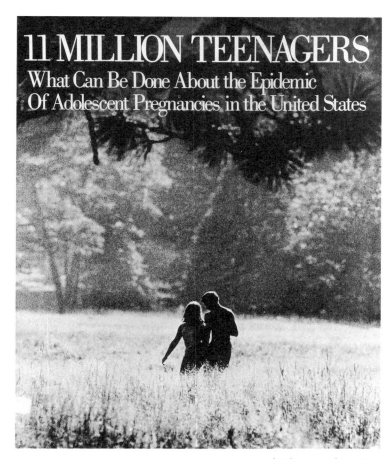

11 MILLION TEENAGERS
What Can Be Done About the Epidemic Of Adolescent Pregnancies in the United States

In 1977, The Alan Guttmacher Institute published 11 Million Teenagers, its first major report on adolescent pregnancy and child-bearing, which helped rouse the nation to a sense of urgency about this devastating tragedy.

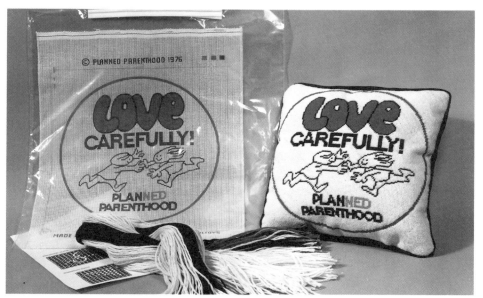

A needlepoint pillow from PPFA's 1976 campaign for sexuality education

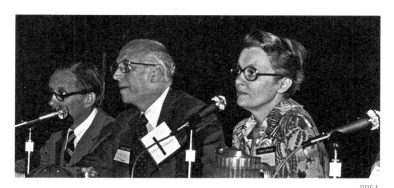

Henrietta H. Marshall, PPFA chairperson from 1975-1978 and acting president from 1976-1977

legislation has strong bipartisan support." He added, "I am confident that by working together — at federal, state and local levels — we can achieve the goal of providing adequate family planning services within the next five years to all those who want them but cannot afford them."

Title X marked an epoch in the tradition of choice. It realized the vision Planned Parenthood had advanced in the 1960s: universal access to family planning services, regardless of age, economic circumstances or place of residence. Title X also called for increased support for research into human reproduction, the development of new contraceptive technology and the creation of an Office of Population Affairs to guide and coordinate government population programs. But its most welcome and visible impact was

on the low-income American women who, for the first time, gained the access to services that other women had. By the end of the decade, more than 5,000 hospitals, public health clinics, neighborhood health centers and women's clinics were offering family planning services that were accessible and affordable.

Title X also fueled an impressive expansion of services offered by Planned Parenthood, especially for low-income women and teens. Over the course of the decade, the number of Planned Parenthood contraceptive patients more than tripled, rising from 345,000 in 1969 to 1,165,000 in 1979. One out of every six of those patients had an income below the federal poverty level — twice the proportion as at the beginning of the decade. One out of three was under 20.

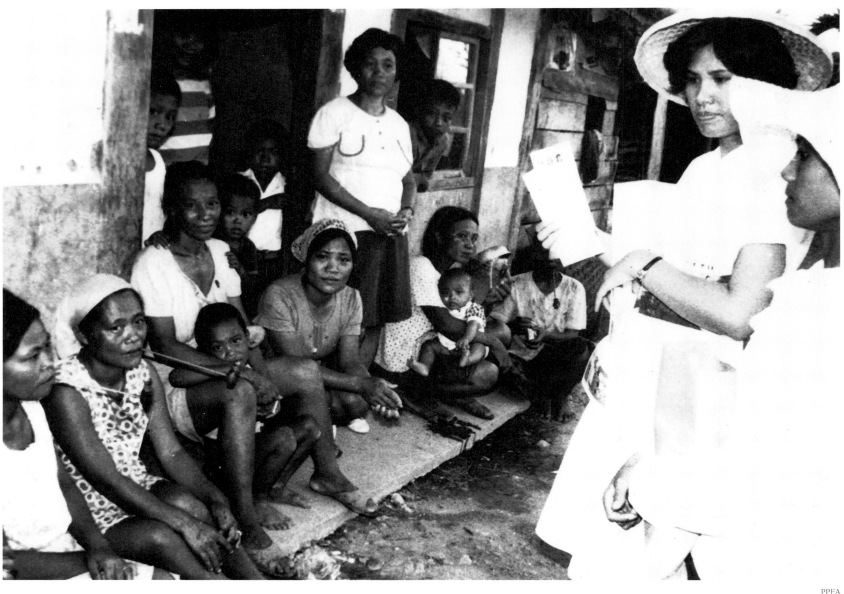

Affiliates launched ambitious programs in sexuality education, often in cooperation with public schools, neighborhood councils, youth-serving organizations and other concerned groups. Imaginative curricula were designed to reach children as young as nine and to help parents talk with their children about sexuality. As new research raised awareness of the extent of adolescent pregnancy and childbearing, Planned Parenthood made education and services for teens a major focus of concern. To attract teens to clinics, affiliates embarked on vigorous publicity campaigns, redesigned their clinic space and created new forms of outreach and service delivery.

During the 1970s, negative publicity about the birth control pill and IUD led to a decline in the number of women choosing these methods and a rise in the number who sought voluntary sterilization. Many Planned Parenthood affiliates opened surgical units to provide outpatient vasectomy and minilaparotomy services. Other new services offered in the 1970s were prenatal care, new forms of infertility treatment and targeted initiatives to attract males — especially teenaged males — to services and involve them in family planning.

In 1971, PPFA added a critical new dimension to its activities. Family Planning International Assistance® (FPIA), the

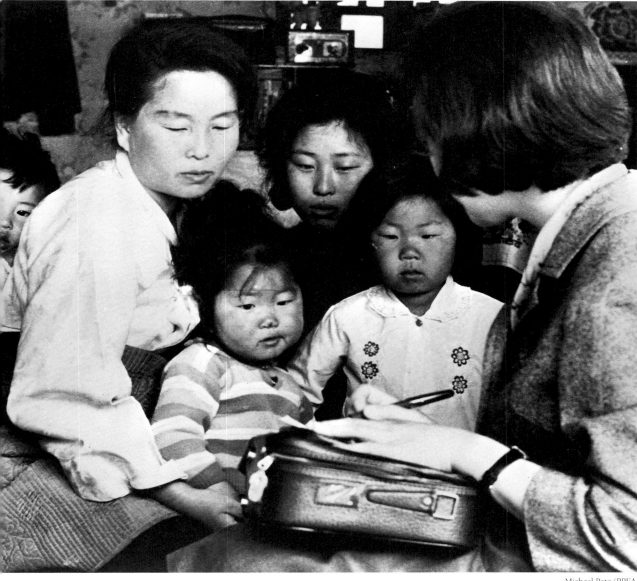

Michael Peto/PPFA

Field workers in programs supported by Family Planning International Assistance (FPIA) offer family planning counseling and services to women in developing countries. Programs for which FPIA provided funding and technical support in the 1970s included: a project that trained village health workers to deliver health services and family planning to hill tribe people in Thailand; a program in Nairobi, Kenya, that promoted breast feeding to enhance child spacing and offered non-hormonal methods of contraception to nursing women; a women's project in Bangladesh that respected the Moslem traditions of this country, where women do not go outside alone, by delivering services to them at home; and a project in Mexico City that established a learning/social center for adolescents incorporating sexuality education and family planning — the first of its kind in Latin America.

organization's international division to support family planning services in developing countries, was formed, at the urgent request of the U.S. Agency for International Development (AID).

While AID's initial request to PPFA was limited to asking the federation to cooperate with Church World Service in shipping contraceptives to mission hospitals, PPFA felt that AID should fund a more comprehensive initiative, including not only the shipping of contraceptives but also program development, training, information and education. AID accepted these arguments and FPIA went on to pioneer many important new concepts in international family planning. It led the way in the development of community-based (non-

clinic) contraceptive distribution projects, involving indigenous villagers in house-to-house distribution of contraceptives. It set precedent by working with local agencies not traditionally active in family planning: labor unions, agricultural cooperatives, youth organizations, Red Cross societies — even Catholic and Muslim organizations. It was the first to incorporate income-generating strategies into family planning project designs. By the end of the 1970s, FPIA had provided over $40 million in assistance to programs designed to become locally controlled and self-supporting in more than 100 countries in Asia, Africa and Latin America.

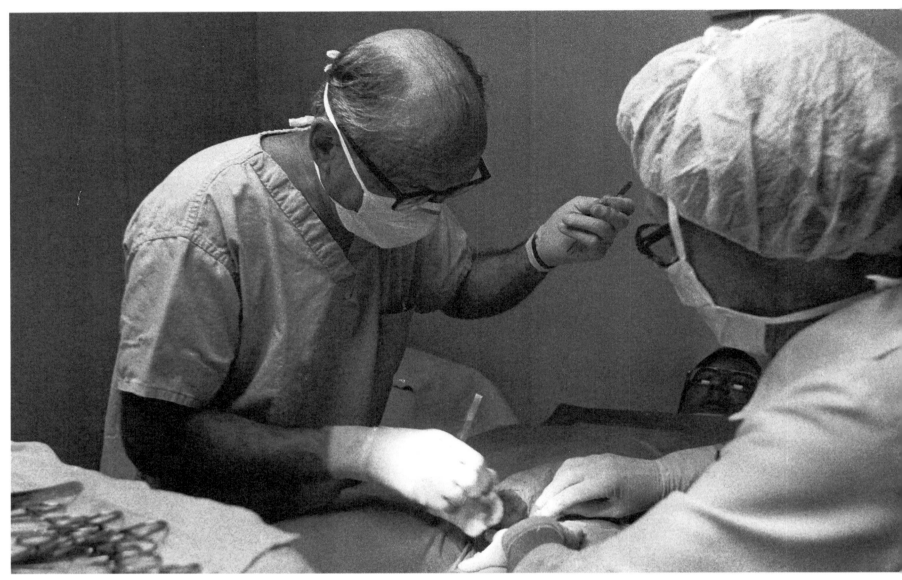

Despite the increased access to contraceptive services in the U.S. and abroad, and for all the distance that had been traveled since Margaret Sanger's arrest, the tragedy of illegal abortion, which first roused Sanger to fight for legal birth control, continued to scar the lives of women and families. Even at this writing, in the 1990s, an estimated 200,000 women worldwide die each year as a result of illegal abortion.

While abortion was opposed by Sanger herself because it led to the deaths of so many women, as the century evolved, it had become a much safer procedure, thanks to major surgical and medical advances. Lobbying of state legislatures to reform abortion laws had begun in earnest after 1959, when the

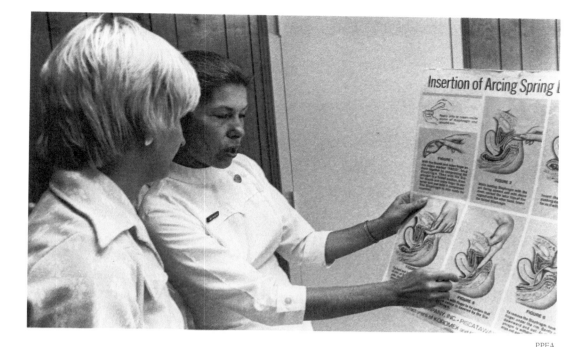

In the 1970s, Title X and other sources of government support drove an enormous expansion of family planning services. Planned Parenthood affiliates launched vigorous campaigns to educate their communities about family planning and encourage the use of services. They also instituted such new services as voluntary sterilization, prenatal care, programs to encourage male involvement and initiatives to provide family planning for disabled people.

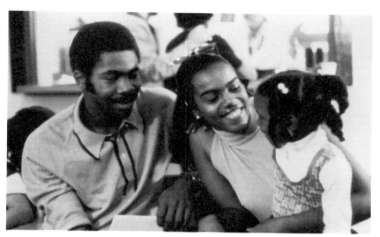

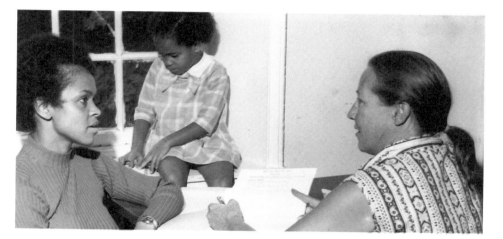

American Law Institute recommended allowing abortion in at least some cases: rape and incest, fetal deformity or grave risk to a woman's mental or physical health. A bill that conformed to the model of the American Law Institute had been signed into law in Colorado in 1967, and another reform law was passed by popular vote in Washington in 1970. In the same year, on April 9, the New York State Legislature passed the most progressive abortion law in the nation, permitting abortion for residents and non-residents of the state alike, for any reason through the 24th week of pregnancy, provided it was performed by a licensed physician.

In July 1970, the Planned Parenthood Center of Syracuse was the first to respond to New York's new law. It started to perform abortions on the first day that the law allowed. Within six months, Planned Parenthood of New York City began providing abortions on a larger scale at its facility in the Bronx.

The opposition, led at first by the Catholic church, organized at once. Picketers massed in front of abortion clinics, screaming epithets at doctors and patients. Anti-abortion organizations sprang up across the country, committed to ensuring that no other state passed a law like New York's. In New York itself, Planned Parenthood affiliates organized a massive statewide educational effort to defeat attempts to overturn the new law.

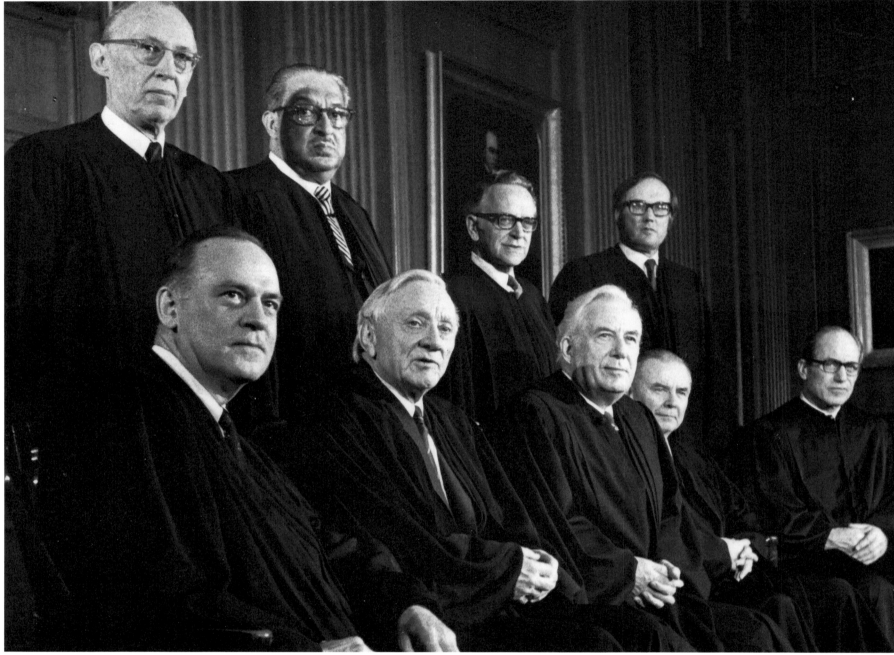

UPI/Bettmann Newsphotos

The Supreme Court that handed down the landmark decision in Roe v. Wade (1973), legalizing abortion nationwide. Seated, from left, are: Potter Stewart, William O. Douglas, Chief Justice Warren E. Burger, William J. Brennan, Jr., and Byron R. White. Standing, from left, are: Lewis F. Powell, Jr., Thurgood Marshall, Harry A. Blackmun and William H. Rehnquist.

On July 1, 1970, the day that New York's liberal new abortion law went into effect, Planned Parenthood of Syracuse became the first affiliate in the nation to offer abortion services. Ellen Fairchild, former executive director, Planned Parenthood of Syracuse, recalled:

"Before the legislature even passed the new law, Dr. Jeff Penfield, the medical director, and I had decided to challenge the state by opening up an abortion clinic. Of course, we never expected the law to be passed. But once it happened, we decided to wait until it took effect on July 1. We did four abortions that first day.

"We had the young and we had the desperate. We even had one whole family of sharecroppers come up from Mississippi because their 13- or 14-year-old girl was pregnant. They had read in the paper that we did abortions and we were the only place they had to turn."

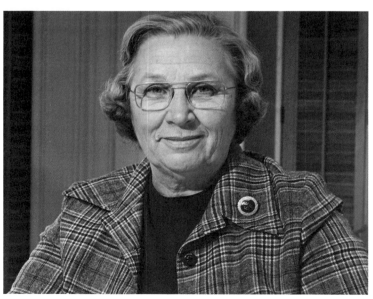

Planned Parenthood Center of Syracuse, Inc.

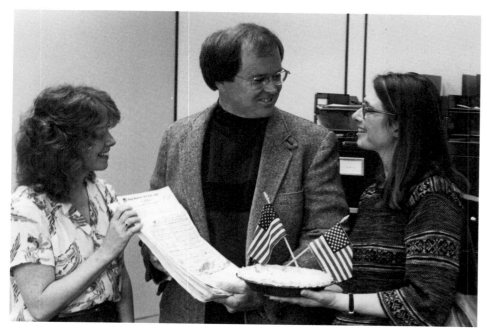

Planned Parenthood affiliates counter anti-choice attacks by reminding legislators and decision-makers that the great majority of Americans support a woman's right to choose. In this 1979 picture, representatives of Planned Parenthood of Santa Cruz County (California), present State Assemblyman Sam Farr with petitions and an apple pie symbolizing their point: "Choice Is as American as Apple Pie."

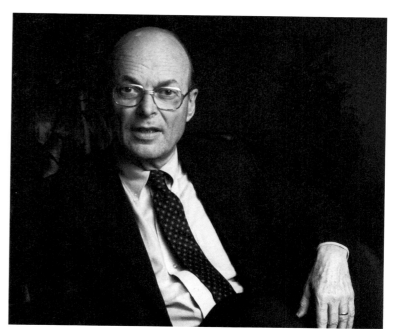

Frederick C. Smith, PPFA chairperson from 1978-1981

A display of educational materials produced by PPFA in the 1970s

There was no going back. In 1973, the Supreme Court's *Roe v. Wade* and *Doe v. Bolton* decisions measured a restrictive Texas statute and a "reform" Georgia statute against constitutional precedent, medical fact and the record of safe and legal abortion compiled in states with the least restrictive laws. By a 7-2 vote, the court ruled that states could no longer interfere with a woman's decision, in consultation with her doctor, to have an abortion in the first three months of pregnancy. After the first trimester, some restrictions were permissible, but not if continued pregnancy threatened the woman's health or life.

With one stroke, the Supreme Court ended the long reign of terror and humiliation against women desperate to end unwanted pregnancy. In a series of subsequent decisions, the court went on to resoundingly affirm *Roe*, striking down requirements that a woman obtain her husband's consent for an abortion and that a teenager obtain her parents' consent.

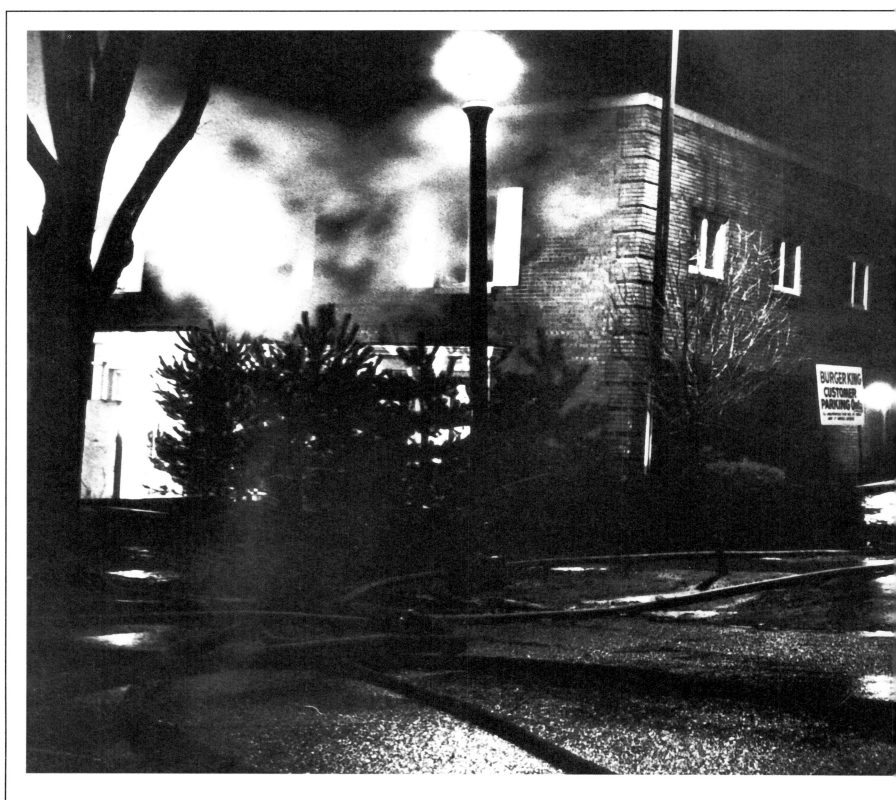

Minnesota Clinic Set Ablaze

Planned Parenthood of Minnesota, founded in 1928, often faced venomous opposition from anti-choice groups. But on February 23, 1977, the hostility turned to criminal violence. The affiliate's St. Paul clinic was set ablaze and by the time the fire was put out, the second floor of the solid brick structure had completely disappeared. Damages totaled over $250,000. A call to a radio station followed — a male voice gloating, "We finally got the abortion clinic."

Since that first fire, there have been three further major arson attacks on the clinic and five bombing attempts. Guns have been fired, cement blocks tossed, windows broken, locks epoxied shut and kidnapping and death threats made against staff and board members — and their children.

Executive Director Tom Webber said, "I'm humbled by what women who have made appointments to terminate unplanned pregnancy will endure. They will wait while people surround their automobiles, throw themselves against their cars, hold bloody fetus signs against the windshield. They'll cry but they don't leave. For whatever complicated reasons women make that difficult decision, they do not change their minds. They will not be deterred, intimidated or threatened. And to watch women endure all this makes one truly appreciate how important the right is. Maybe that's why we stay here."

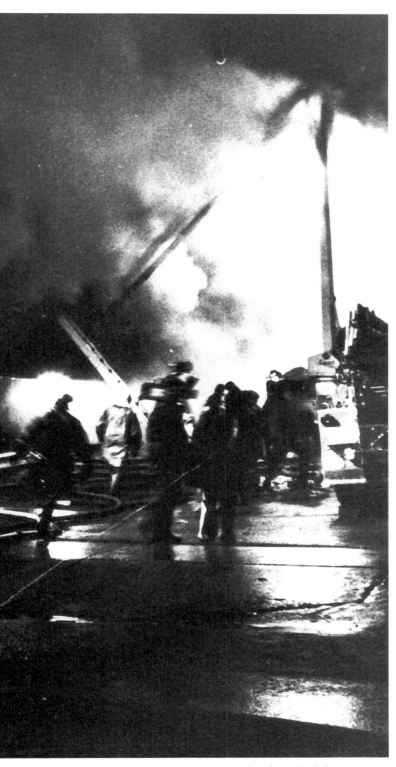

Planned Parenthood of Minnesota, Inc.

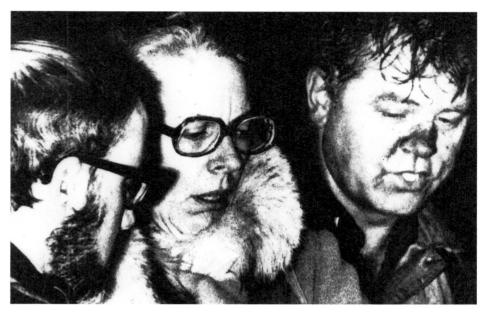

Planned Parenthood of Minnesota, Inc.

Shown on the night of the fire are (from left) Tom Webber, executive director; Kitt Briggs, board president; and a firefighter.

Nationwide, the Catholic church and other opposition groups applied massive pressure to deny women their new-won right. In 1976, opponents of choice pushed through Congress the first version of the Hyde Amendment, barring the use of Medicaid funds to pay for abortion in all circumstances except when a woman's life was endangered or she was the victim of rape or incest. Picketers (euphemistically called "sidewalk counselors") began efforts to physically stop women from entering clinics, sometimes punching and kicking them. A wave of arson attacks and bombings destroyed clinics and terrorized patients and staff.

It might have been understandable if, at that point, Planned Parenthood had quietly retreated from the front lines. But in 1978, the PPFA board chose as its new president Faye Wattleton, former executive director of the Planned Parenthood Association of Miami Valley, in Dayton, Ohio. At 34 the youngest person, the first African-American and the first woman since Sanger to lead Planned Parenthood, Wattleton took office determined to push the tradition of choice to the next frontier.

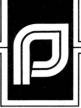

THE 1980s: IN THE LINE OF FIRE

"As president of Planned Parenthood, I have strongly opposed the abuse and misuse of power by traditional institutions and have certainly not had a mind to capitulate simply because the president of the United States said so."

—Faye Wattleton in a 1991 interview

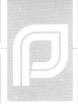

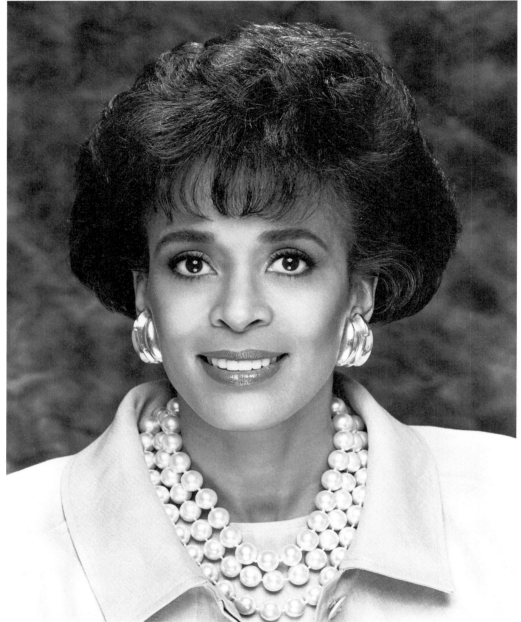

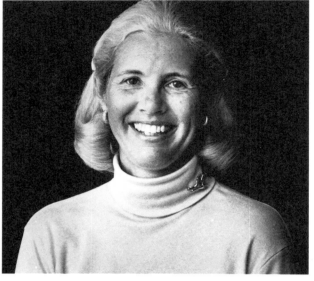

Jean Mahoney, PPFA chairperson 1981-1984

PPFA

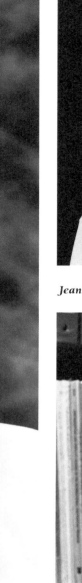

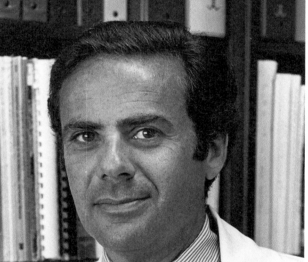

Allan Rosenfield, M.D., PPFA chairperson from 1984-1986

PPFA

Eric Stephen Jacobs

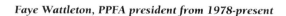

Faye Wattleton, PPFA president from 1978-present

The 1980s, the era of Ronald Reagan's presidency, was breezily called by the White House "a new morning in America." But the Reagan administration's disregard of civil liberties and ruthless cutbacks in basic services for the poor, disabled and elderly made it a cheerless dawn for millions. Since then, George Bush's succession to the White House has let in scant new sunlight.

Although President Reagan took the oath of office with a pledge to end government intrusion in people's lives, his social-issues agenda appeared designed to do the opposite.

This agenda expressed Reagan's indebtedness to the New Right, a loose coalition of right-wing and extremist groups that formed in the late 1970s and whose agendas bore a striking resemblance to the anti-vice movement of Anthony Comstock a century earlier. The chief common ground of these extremists was opposition to abortion. In its effort to drive women back to the dangers of enforced childbearing and illegal abortion that marked the early part of the century, the New Right has made strenuous efforts to put an end to government-funded family planning services and to overturn *Roe v. Wade*.

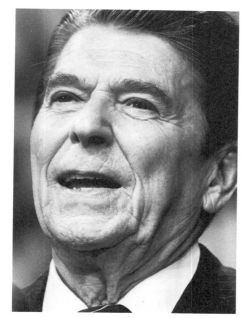

As president, Ronald Reagan actively sought to curtail and restrict access to family planning services and to eliminate the right to safe, legal abortion.

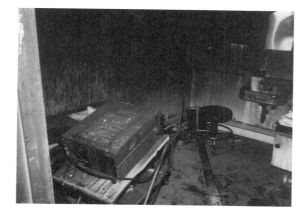

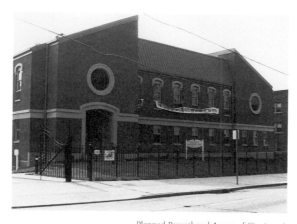

These photos show the headquarters of Planned Parenthood Association of Cincinnati as it looked after being bombed by anti-choice fanatics in December 1985 and the rebuilt clinic opened in 1987 at a new location with the support of the community.

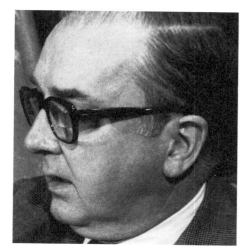

Fanatical views and manipulative political tactics marked Senator Jesse Helms (Republican-North Carolina) as the Anthony Comstock of the late 20th century. A New Right stalwart, he authored much of the anti-family planning, anti-choice legislation of the 1980s.

The Impact of Title X in the 1980s

Virtually all the nation's family planning agencies depend to some extent on public funding sources to provide services for low-income women and teens, and Title X is the mainstay of the system of public funding. In 1983, publicly funded family planning agencies provided services to an estimated 4.1 million people a year at 5,100 clinic sites. Nearly one in four American women using contraceptives each year (exclusive of sterilization) obtained services from a publicly funded provider. The typical client was young, had a low or marginal income as defined by the federal poverty index and did not yet have children. Sixty-three percent were white. Young women under 20 represented one-third of all patients.

Without government support, an estimated 1.2 million additional unintended pregnancies would have occurred each year during the 1980s, resulting in approximately 516,000 abortions and 509,000 unwanted births. Taxpayers saved $4.40 for every public dollar spent to provide birth control for women who might not otherwise have had access to contraception.

But public opinion polls proved that the great majority of Americans remained strongly supportive of accessible family planning services and safe and legal abortion. They respected Planned Parenthood as an ethical service provider that would uphold their cherished tradition of choice. As Planned Parenthood's president, Faye Wattleton took that public trust seriously. In the words of a *Time* reporter, she "took off the white gloves and became one of the nation's most vocal and aggressive advocates" of reproductive rights.

Wattleton moved quickly to reorganize the structure of the national organization, to establish a strong lobbying presence in Washington, to mobilize grass-roots support through a nationwide public impact campaign, to launch an aggressive program of litigation in federal and state courts and to implement nationwide, hard-hitting advertising programs. Within a few years, the media came to acknowledge her as a forceful presence and a master strategist and spokesperson, who had repositioned Planned Parenthood as a leader in the fight for reproductive freedom.

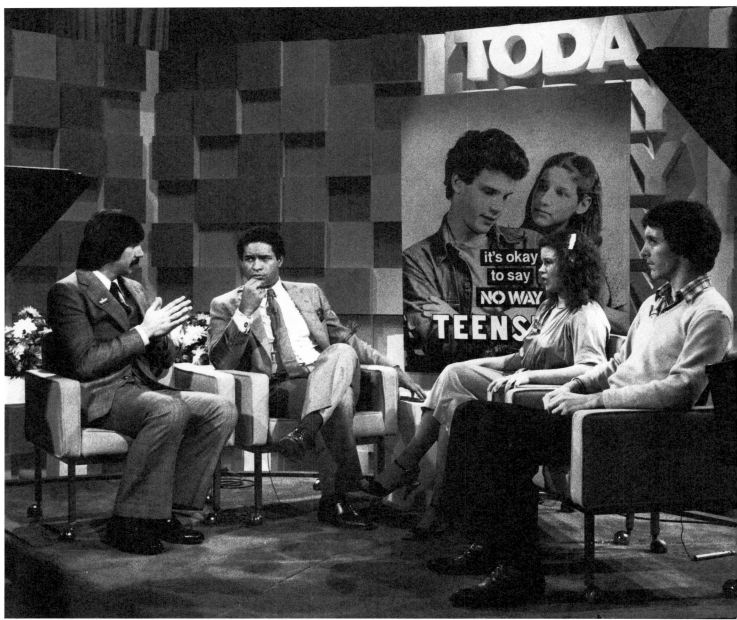

Counseling teens about sexuality was the theme of the nationally televised "Today" show on January 15, 1982. Seated with host Bryant Gumbel before a wall-sized blow-up of a Planned Parenthood pamphlet are (far left) Tony Silvestrin, staff educator for Planned Parenthood of Seattle-King County (Washington), and (far right) Lora Rinehart and Gary Conely, Planned Parenthood peer counselors.

Raimondo Borea/PPFA

Anne Saunier, PPFA chairperson from 1986-1989

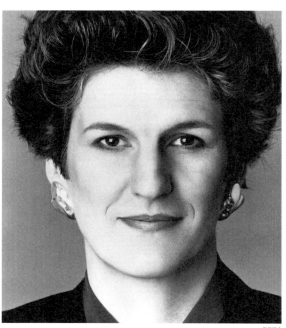

PPFA

At a time when withdrawal of government support put pressure on many nonprofit organizations to curtail services, Wattleton spoke out resoundingly in favor of expanding access to reproductive health care for those most in need — the poor and the young. She took the offensive in renewing Planned Parenthood's commitment to informed, comprehensive, age-appropriate sexuality education for every American — not only to combat the tragedies of unwanted pregnancy and abortion but, in the tradition of Margaret Sanger, to help people accept their sexuality as a normal and healthy part of life.

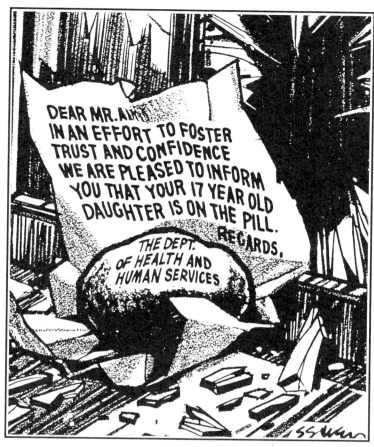

Cartoonist David Seavey thought the Reagan administration's proposed notice to parents when teens obtained contraception would be about as welcome as a rock hurled through a window. His cartoon was one of the hundreds of media responses generated by Planned Parenthood's successful campaign to get the "squeal rule" overturned.

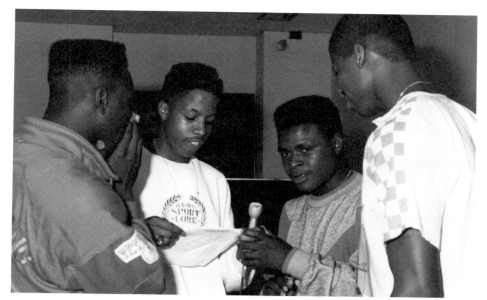

Creative and sensitive approaches to attract teens to clinics continued to be a major focus of Planned Parenthood in the 1980s. In this photo, high school students Antoine Sipp, Derrick Grey, Charles Howleit and Robert Murphy audition their rapping for a public service announcement by Planned Parenthood of Chicago.

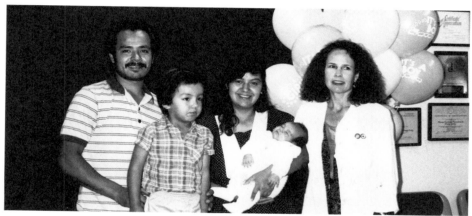

The prenatal care program of Planned Parenthood/Orange & San Bernardino Counties (Santa Ana, California) serves mostly Spanish-speaking families. The program was launched because 2,000 pregnant women in the area were being refused services at public agencies each year. Here Kathy Grossman (right), prenatal care coordinator, joins a celebration of the first baby born in the program.

Reinforcing these national efforts were Planned Parenthood affiliates' battles to preserve and extend reproductive choice through campaigns in their states and communities. They lobbied, sponsored symposia and other community forums, educated decision-makers and the media, advertised, filed lawsuits and forged coalitions with other community groups. They even used humor and wit to exploit the rising harassment and violence against clinics — Pledge-A-Picket campaigns in many local areas raised thousands of dollars by asking donors to pledge a specific amount for each anti-choice picket showing up at a clinic on a given day.

These determined initiatives proved key to the defeat of New Right efforts, led by Ronald Reagan, to defund and thereby destroy Title X. While funding for Title X declined, the program remained a vital source of family planning services and other reproductive health care for four million low-income women and teens every year.

Planned Parenthood also led the successful grass-roots organizing effort to defeat the Reagan administration's "squeal rule," an attempt to drive teens away from Title X- funded clinics by mandating parental notification when teens received prescription services. In summer 1983, two federal courts threw out the rule, denouncing the administration's arguments in its favor as "fatuous" and "mere sophistry."

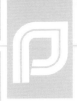

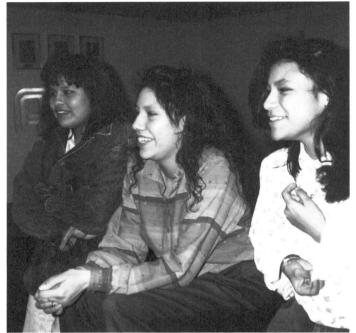

Teens from Planned Parenthood of Central Oklahoma's TIPI (Teen Indian Peer Improvement) performance troupe. TIPI's video, "Circle of Life: Wellness and Sexuality," was the first in the nation to address preventing pregnancy and HIV infections among Native American teens.

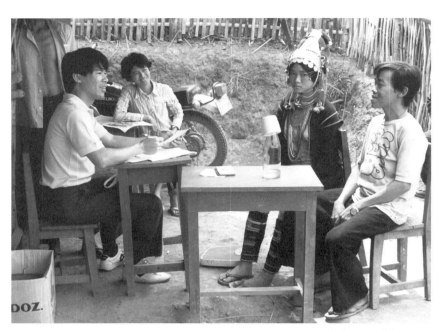

A hill tribe couple in Thailand receives family planning counseling from the staff member of a project supported by PPFA's international division, Family Planning International Assistance (FPIA). From 1972, when FPIA began providing support, through 1989, the value of FPIA assistance to international programs totaled over $224 million. In 1989 alone, the projects it funded provided contraceptive services to 1.6 million clients.

In 1986, a government-sponsored evaluation commented that FPIA had "demonstrated dedication, leadership, creativity, courage and above all success under difficult LDC [less developed countries] conditions."

The elimination of U.S. government funding for FPIA meant the end of family planning projects in Thailand, Pakistan, Turkey, Indonesia, Sri Lanka and Haiti and the withdrawal of support for new projects in India, Nepal, Cameroon and Kenya. It is anticipated at this writing that AID's decision will result in the loss of contraceptive services to at least 500,000 individuals.

But while the Reagan administration was temporarily blocked from imposing its anti-family-planning, anti-abortion policies at home, it succeeded in exporting them abroad. The "Mexico City policy" (named after the 1984 international conference at which the policy was announced) is a clause added to the contracts that AID signs with international agencies. It bars these agencies from underwriting any overseas family planning program that performs, advocates, refers or counsels women about abortion — even when those programs are operated entirely by local grantees in countries where such activities are legal and paid for by private funds. In the late 1980s and early 1990s, this anti-choice position led to the

defunding of many major international family planning agencies, including the International Planned Parenthood Federation and Planned Parenthood's international division, FPIA.

Most ominously, Reagan, while in office, stacked the federal courts, including the Supreme Court, with ultra-conservatives hostile to the fundamental guarantees of *Roe v. Wade*. In 1989, the court ruled on the case of *Webster v. Reproductive Health Services*, which challenged a law passed in the Missouri Legislature that posed a host of restrictions on access to abortion. In an unprecedented departure from previous rulings, the court upheld portions of the law and hinted that it might be ready to reconsider the reasoning

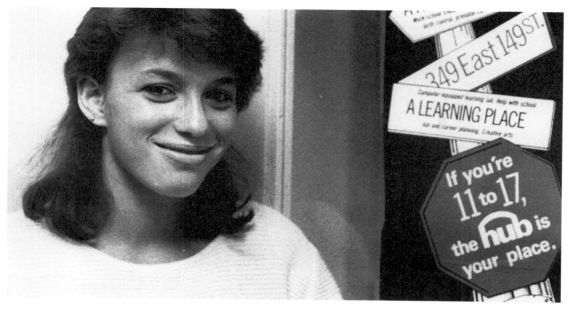

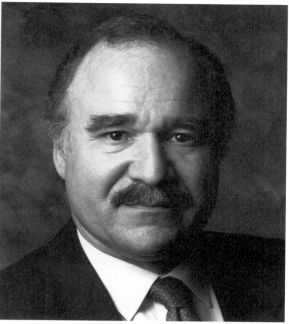

Planned Parenthood of New York City

Shown here is a teen client of Planned Parenthood of New York City's (PPNYC's) Hub Center, which provides comprehensive services, including family planning, to women in the South Bronx, the poorest congressional district in the U.S., with one of the highest rates of teen childbearing.

The Hub's medical director, Dr. Irving Rust, was the lead plaintiff in the U.S. Supreme Court suit challenging the Reagan and Bush administrations' "gag rule," which bars clinics from counseling or referring clients for abortions as long as they receive Title X funds. Rust was motivated to go to court in part by memories of his 1960s hospital residency in New York City, when abortions were illegal. He recalled, "We basically stayed in the operating room and did D&C's on septic or incomplete abortions — 15 or 20 of them a day, many on women who were near death."

The gag rule, Rust believes, threatens to bring back those days for poor women and teens who depend on publicly funded clinics. He said, "Under the gag rule, a pregnant woman who comes to us is supposed to be referred for prenatal care. Period. We are not supposed to mention abortion even if she asks. We are just supposed to respond, if asked, that we do not consider abortion a method of family planning and can only refer her to a clinic that does not do abortions."

For the sake of the 5,000 women and teens, many of them desperately poor, who come to the Hub every year, Rust vows, "I will not be gagged."

PPFA

Kenneth C. Edelin, M.D., PPFA chairperson from 1989-present, is a gynecologist and obstetrician who is one of the nation's leading advocates for sexuality education, access to family planning services, and reproductive rights. The former director of obstetrics and gynecology at Boston City Hospital, Edelin also serves as associate dean for student and minority affairs at Boston University School of Medicine.

that had formed the basis of *Roe* and nearly two decades of progress in reproductive rights.

In 1990, the court further restricted access to abortion for teenagers with its decisions in *Hodgson v. Minnesota and Ohio v. Akron Center for Reproductive Health.*

One year later, the Supreme Court — its right-wing majority further enlarged by President George Bush — shocked the nation again by upholding the Reagan and Bush administrations' "gag rule," which bars staff in Title X-funded clinics from giving pregnant women information about abortion — even if they ask for the information.

These alarming attacks against reproductive rights have accelerated the activism of Planned Parenthood and the pro-choice majority across the U.S. In April 1989, in anticipation of the court's ruling in the *Webster* case, an estimated half-million marchers created the largest pro-choice demonstration in history in Washington, D.C. In November, after the ruling, a nationally coordinated day of rallies drew an unprecedented two million Americans who participated in more than 1,000 pro-choice events. And in 1991, after the "gag rule" decision, a campaign by Planned Parenthood and a tremendous outcry by Americans spurred the U.S. Congress to consider legislation that would affirm the obligation and longstanding practice of Title X- funded clinics to counsel pregnant women about all their legal options.

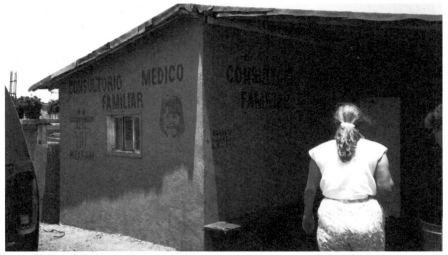

Planned Parenthood of San Diego and Riverside Counties

In 1986, Planned Parenthood of San Diego & Riverside Counties (PPSDRC) California, pioneered a bi-national initiative. It teamed up with MexFam, the International Planned Parenthood Federation affiliate in Mexico, to open a constellation of low-cost family planning clinics in fast-growing Tijuana, Mexico. Mark Salo, executive director, explained, "The human need for family planning doesn't end at the border. It's universal. We have to be innovative to find responses because the needs present themselves." Financed in part by PPSDRC, the clinics are adapted from a model developed by MexFam that allows them to become self-sufficient after the first few years.

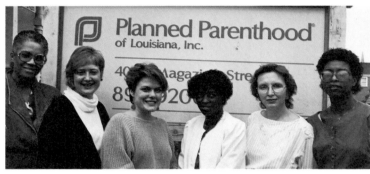

Planned Parenthood of Louisiana, Inc.

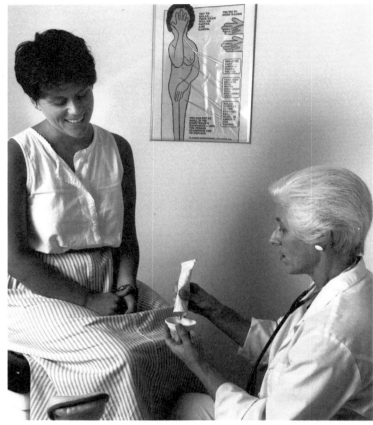

Cathy Blaivas/PPFA

In the 1980s, the use of nurse practitioners to provide reproductive health care services to healthy women became standard practice in Planned Parenthood clinics.

The first Planned Parenthood affiliate in Louisiana opened its doors in New Orleans in May 1984. Shown at left are: Ruby Phillip; Julie Redman, director of education; Terri Bartlett, executive director; Jacqueline Tate; Kathleen Martin; and Phillipa Wells Harrison.

Essential to Planned Parenthood's mission as this activism is, in the words of Anne Saunier, PPFA chairperson from 1986 to 1989, "Planned Parenthood is first and foremost a service provider; and furthering that mission of service is the single purpose of our advocacy efforts." As a service provider, Planned Parenthood grew and thrived throughout the decade. In 1989, 1.6 million Americans participated in sexuality education sessions led by Planned Parenthood staff and volunteers in every imaginable community setting — schools, hospitals, group homes, community centers, country fairs, prisons. Another 1.7 million Americans turned to Planned Parenthood for contraceptive services — a 45 percent increase over the previous decade.

Affiliates showed resourcefulness and sensitivity in attracting new populations to services. In Oklahoma City, Planned Parenthood of Central Oklahoma offered "Straight Talk" programs in which trained sexuality educators facilitated discussions among young adolescents and parents. In Boise, Planned Parenthood of Idaho held mother/daughter workshops to promote responsible decision-making. In Milwaukee County, Planned Parenthood of Wisconsin organized a Life Options Coalition of community groups concerned with reducing the rate of teen pregnancy in the state.

Planned Parenthood of South Palm Beach and Broward Counties (Florida) showed an original 15-minute filmstrip on family planning

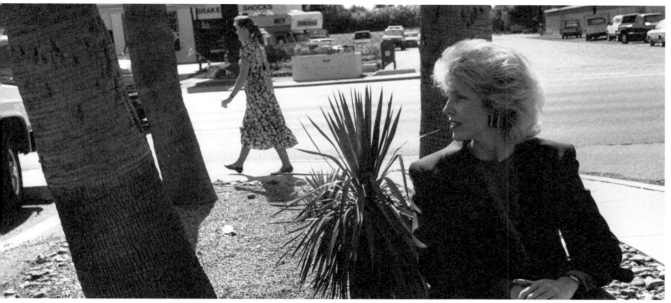

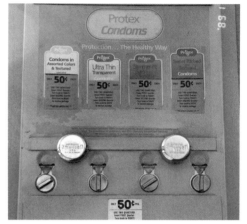

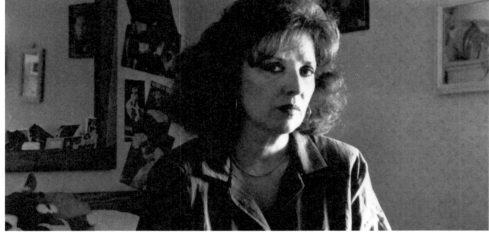

in English, Spanish and Creole as part of a refugee resettlement program in Fort Lauderdale. The Planned Parenthood Center of Austin (Texas) helped organize an effort by local Latino gang members to create a rap video and a pregnancy prevention/safe sex mural.

As public confidence in Planned Parenthood continued to grow, the range of services people received increased as well. For example, Planned Parenthood Shasta-Diablo (Walnut Creek, California), which expanded from five to 12 centers during the 1980s, offered, in addition to gynecological check-ups and family planning care, the following services:

- testing and treatment for sexually transmitted diseases in both women and men

- a pioneering program in HIV testing and counseling, which became a model for the state of California

- ultrasonography

- abortions up to 16 weeks of pregnancy

- colposcopy for early treatment of dysplasia to prevent cervical cancer

- male and female sterilization

- infertility treatment and counseling

- midlife services, including estrogen replacement therapy

- prenatal care

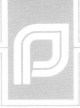

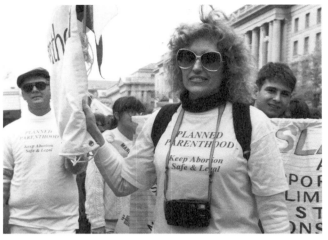
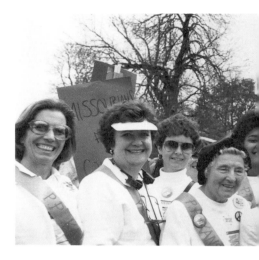

Joan Marcus/PPFA

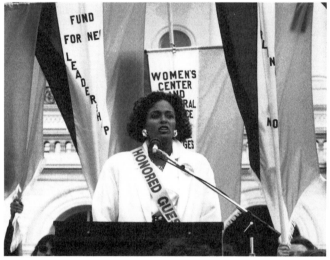

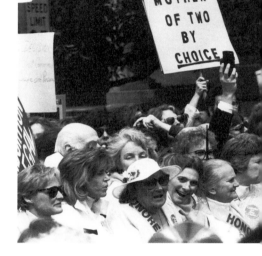

Art Stein/PPFA

In a move that has proven both cost-effective and pleasing to patients, affiliates in the 1980s expanded their use of specially trained nurses — "nurse practitioners" — and physician's assistants to provide the majority of non-surgical services. While physicians continue to supervise the delivery of all medical care and deal directly with cases involving serious pathology, by the end of the decade, nurse practitioners were providing about 75 percent of all direct patient care offered at Planned Parenthood affiliates. Their sensitivity and expertise won wide approval from clients and health professionals and served as a model for other health care agencies.

Strikingly, in the face of continuing harassment and violence against family planning and abortion clinics, more affiliates than ever put themselves on the line providing abortion services. In the course of the decade, the number of affiliates offering this service increased by 32 percent, to a total of 53. Kenneth C. Edelin, M.D., PPFA chairperson since 1989, explained why:

"More and more affiliates want to offer abortion services because they have a real commitment to this issue. This is the line that has been drawn in the sand. We recognize that if the opposition is successful in outlawing abortion, they will come after contraception next."

While Planned Parenthood has continued to heighten its visibility on challenging issues, it has also endured as one of the most cherished and respected not-for-profit organizations. In a 1989 Gallup poll, 82 percent of Americans had a favorable opinion

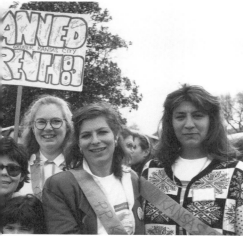

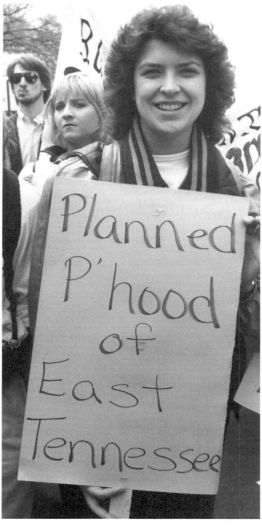

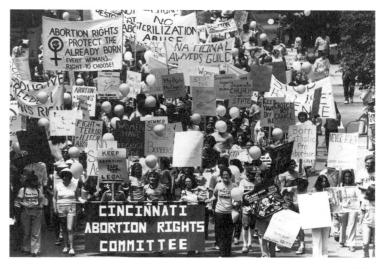

PPFA

Llewellyn W. Bensfield

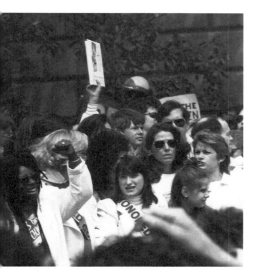

PPFA

Joan Marcus/PPFA

Joan Marcus/PPFA

of PPFA, with only two nonprofit organizations — the American Cancer Society and the League of Women Voters — rated more highly.

As the decade ended, Planned Parenthood deepened its commitment to preserve reproductive freedom by founding a new political arm, the Planned Parenthood Action Fund. Contributions to the Action Fund, a 501(c)(4) organization, are not tax deductible, leaving the fund free to carry on unlimited lobbying and limited electoral campaign activity. It can publicize the pro-choice or anti-choice records of candidates and conduct voter education and identification drives, among other activities. The Action Fund is an important asset in translating the deep belief in choice that characterizes mainstream America into an even more effective political movement.

Despite the relentless attacks on reproductive freedom that marked the Reagan years, the 1980s were a decade in which Planned Parenthood and the tradition it stands for achieved new levels of strength and support. To quote Faye Wattleton:

"As we persevered in our efforts to prevent the need for abortion through greater access to contraception and educational services, we also helped to preserve the right of all American women to safe and legal abortion, a necessary element of reproductive choice. The ongoing support of the majority of Americans will ensure our continued success."

Planned Parenthood entered the 1990s with confidence that the tradition of choice would withstand any further assaults, and that greater victories lay ahead.

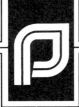

THE 1990s: FROM THESE ROOTS

"It is not enough to look backward with pride, justified as that pride may be. We must look forward with hope and confidence, too. The real lesson of the past is that it shows us what can be done for the future."

—Margaret Sanger

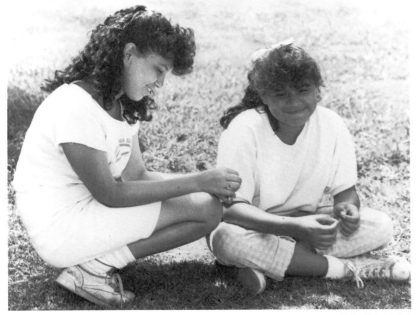

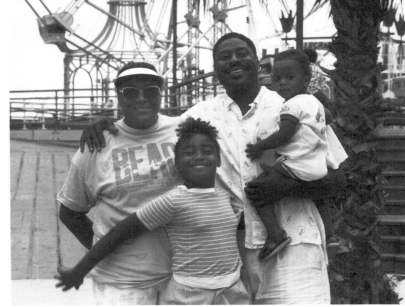

Cathy Blaivas/PPFA

Cathy Blaivas/PPFA

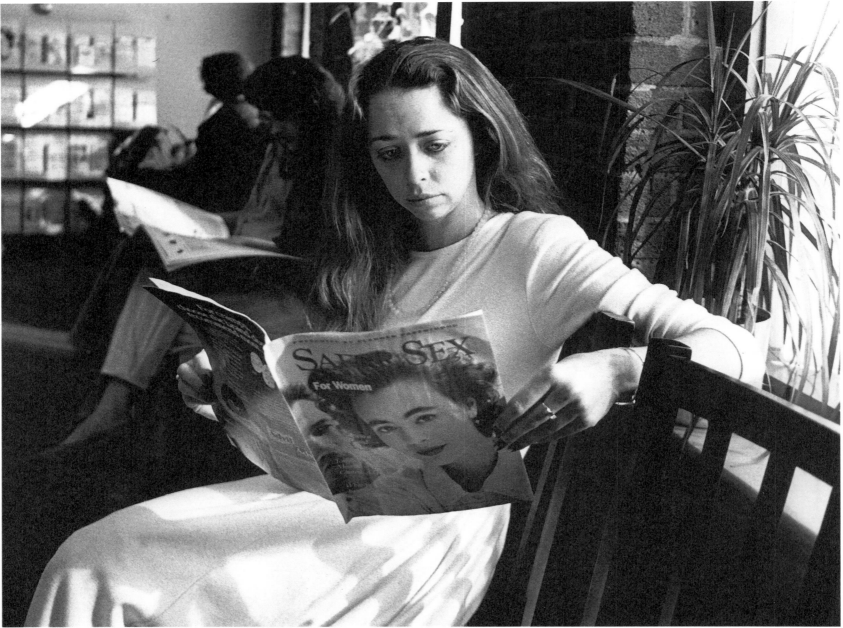

Gale Zucker

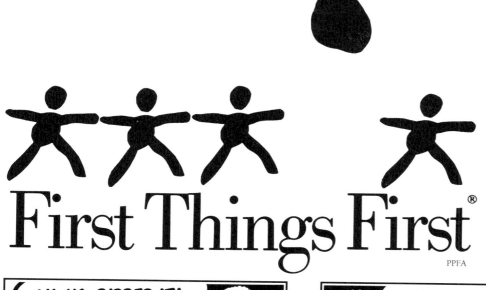

First Things First®

PPFA

Since the 1970s, PPFA has worked to place the tragedy of teen pregnancy and childbearing on the nation's list of priorities. In the 1990s, Planned Parenthood is tapping that concern to bring about actual change through a new, comprehensive, nationwide initiative: First Things First.®

First Things First aims to reduce by half the number of adolescents who become pregnant and give birth by the year 2000. It provides a framework and concrete support for local initiatives in sexuality education, clinical services and community organization.

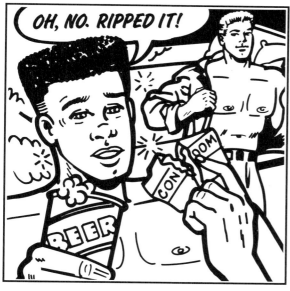

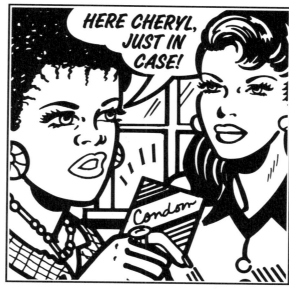

Planned Parenthood's AIDS prevention pamphlet targeted to sexually active teenagers was published in 1990. Called " It Can't Happen to Me!—True Stories About AIDS," it is designed to help teens understand that they, too, are at risk for HIV infections.

Copyright Robert Dale 1990

In the 1990s, an era of astonishing technological advances, lasers map illness in the human body and satellite-borne telescopes peer into distant galaxies. Yet poverty, unwanted childbirth and ravaging diseases, including AIDS, crush the lives of millions in the U.S. and abroad. A global recession threatens to intensify their pain — and to strike particularly hard against women and children, who are the great majority of the poor. To ensure a future in which access to reproductive health care and reproductive choice is an unquestioned right, Planned Parenthood faces grave challenges in the coming years.

The family planning movement has achieved great progress since 1965, when the U.S. Supreme Court's *Griswold* decision

assured at least married couples the right to practice birth control. Since that time, the percentage of unintended births (babies born when their mothers didn't want a child at all, or didn't want a child at that particular time) has declined by almost half nationwide.

But American women in the 1990s still experience more than three million unintended pregnancies each year. Nearly half of them end in abortion. Teenagers account for almost one million of the unintended pregnancies in this country each year and half of them choose abortion.

Planned Parenthood is committed to a broad array of initiatives to change this reality. Chief among its priorities is the promotion of open and responsible discussions of sexuality in the home, schools, community and media.

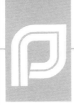

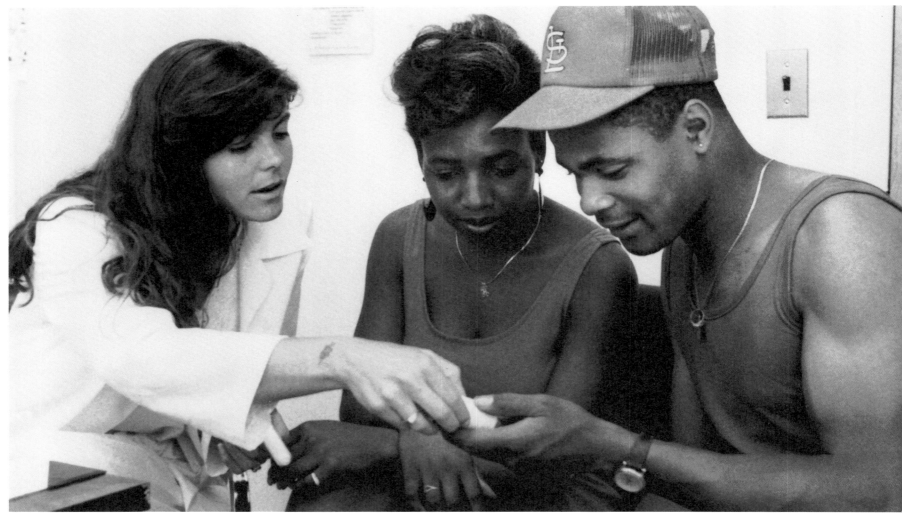

Cathy Blaivas/PPFA

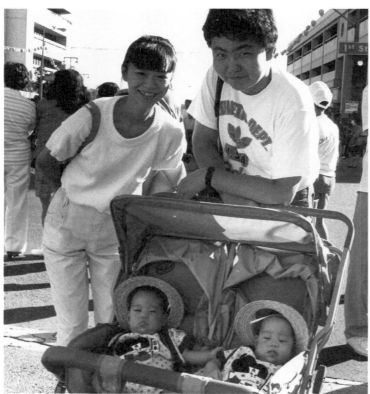

Cathy Blaivas/PPFA

Many American adults, confused and embarrassed by their own sexuality, hesitate to discuss sexual matters with their children. And fewer than 10 percent of all young people receive timely, comprehensive sexuality education in the schools. The lack of information and education robs them of the reproductive choice that should be their birthright. But teaching children how their bodies work, how to avoid risky behavior and how to plan for their futures is as fundamental as teaching them how to read or add. And helping people of all ages understand their sexuality and plan their families is as fundamentally life-giving as assisting them to earn a living or prevent disease. These basic truths must be acknowledged on the nation's agenda in the 1990s.

As opponents of family planning continue attempts to curtail or eliminate Title X— the

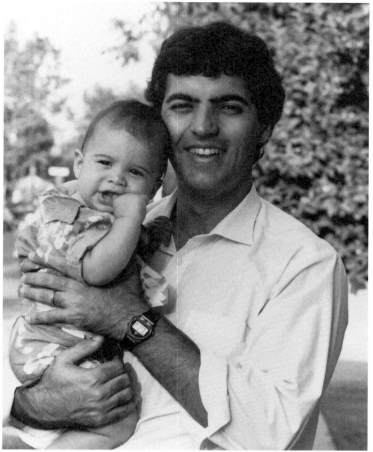

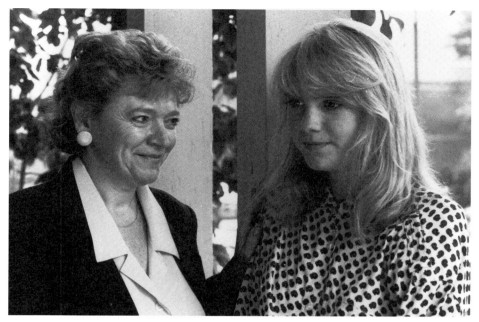

Cathy Blaivas/PPFA

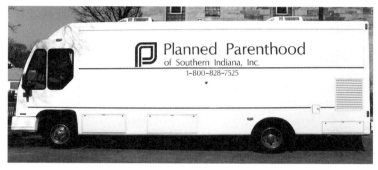

Planned Parenthood of Southern Indiana, Inc.

Planned Parenthood is the trusted source of reliable information and quality health care for women and men of all ages, backgrounds and income levels.

Cathy Blaivas/PPFA

principal guarantee of accessible, affordable family planning services in the U.S. — Planned Parenthood remains vigilant in safeguarding its survival. Planned Parenthood is also working to ensure that FPIA and other international agencies can continue to support the provision of family planning services for people in the world's poorest countries, where reproductive health care is as vital to survival as food and water.

In the 1990s, the U.S., for all its technological superiority and wealth, is failing its people when it comes to providing the best and widest choices of birth control. Americans today have fewer birth control options than do people in many European countries and even some developing countries. Decades after the start of the birth control revolution, the only reversible method for men remains the

condom — making it more difficult for men to share responsibility for contraception.

Under the Reagan and Bush administrations, government support and funding for contraceptive research — one of the cornerstone provisions of Title X— has diminished. The prohibitive costs of researching and developing new contraceptives, combined with the fear of defending against expensive lawsuits even for methods that have proven safe, has led private industry to withdraw from the field. Finally, the vocal opposition of the anti-choice movement (which seems unable or unwilling to see that the only way to prevent abortion is to prevent unintended pregnancy) has contributed to a climate discouraging to the introduction of new methods.

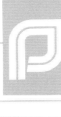

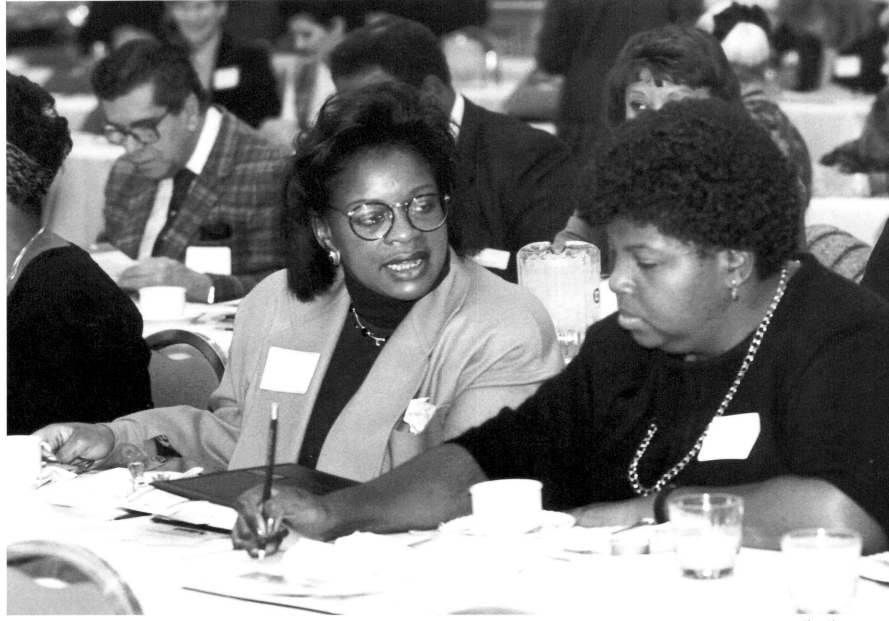

Photo Ideas

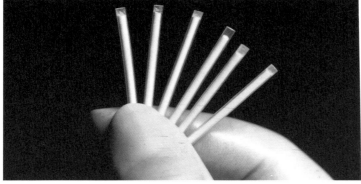

The Population Council

A bright spot in the area of contraceptive technology appeared in 1991, when the U.S. Food and Drug Administration gave its approval for the first time in 25 years to a new birth control method, Norplant®. Norplant was developed by the Population Council under the guidance of Dr. Sheldon Segal. It is a familiar contraceptive formula that uses a novel method of delivery: Tiny progestin-releasing rods are inserted just under the skin of the upper arm, protecting a woman from unwanted pregnancy for five years. As soon as approval was announced, Planned Parenthood affiliates began training health care professionals to offer this method to women.

Planned Parenthood's Campaign for New Birth Control is countering that opposition. It is pressing to heighten appreciation of the need for new birth control options, to make contraceptive research and development a national priority, to encourage public funding and incentives for the development of new technology and to streamline the process through which new methods are introduced to the public.

Finally, in the coming decade, Planned Parenthood dedicates itself with renewed energy and optimism to eliminating the last barriers to reproductive choice. It will

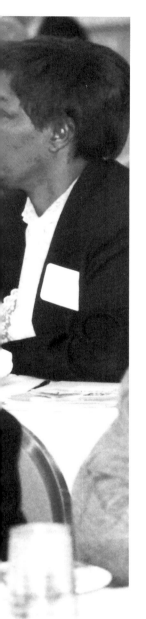

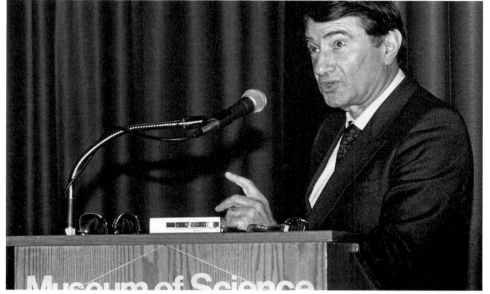

Campaign for New Birth Control
(Near left) Dr. Etienne-Emile Baulieu addresses participants at a PPFA-sponsored conference on new birth control in Boston, February 12, 1990; (far left) participants at another conference in the series, held in Chicago, March 15, 1990.

Baulieu led the development of RU 486, a compound that, when given with prostaglandin, appears to be a safe and effective alternative to early surgical abortion. Manufactured by the French company, Roussel-Uclaf, RU 486 was introduced in France in 1988. By avoiding the necessity for invasive procedures, it has the potential to make abortion in the U.S. a more truly private decision between a woman and her doctor and to prevent thousands of deaths from illegal, often self-induced abortions in the developing world.

Marilyn Humphries

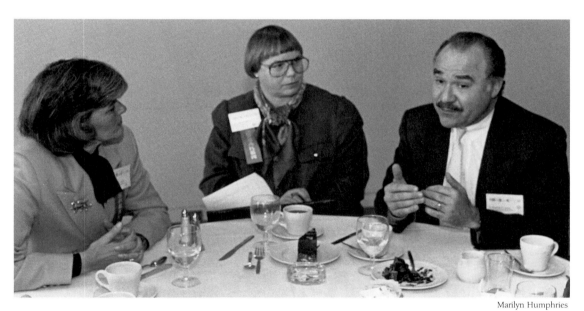

Dr. Kenneth Edelin, PPFA chairperson, makes a point to Nicki Nichols Gamble, executive director of Planned Parenthood League of Massachusetts (seated at his right), and Representative Patricia Schroeder (Democrat-Colorado), during the PPFA new birth control conference in Boston.

Marilyn Humphries

continue to urge Congress to translate the majority support for safe and legal abortion and unrestricted access to family planning services into the law of the land, and to halt anti-choice efforts to undercut our precious freedom of choice in matters of childbearing.

In 1991, Faye Wattleton said:

"Seventy-five years ago, Margaret Sanger planted the roots of our movement in political change. She referred to the fight for reproductive freedom as 'the fundamental revolt...for woman, the key to the temple of liberty.' She risked everything, including prison, for that revolt. She refused to tolerate oppression and she refused to

compromise. Now more than ever, we must remember these roots."

From the roots Sanger planted in 1916, the tradition of choice has grown like a great forest, protecting and nourishing all who live within its shade. Reproductive freedom is no longer a rare plant, the secret of a wealthy few. It has become a familiar habitat for millions, making possible life, health and happiness that past generations only dreamed of.

Planned Parenthood's commitment, in its 75th year, is to extend the gift of this mighty tradition to all.

Afterword: The Early History of Birth Control

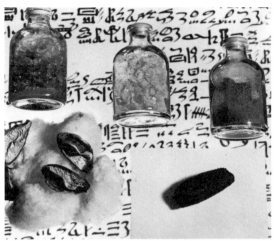

Ortho Pharmaceutical (Canada) Ltd.

A re-creation of an early Egyptian contraceptive tampon (right), displayed with the ingredients used to make it: fine wool, acacia, dates and honey

Nearly every civilization has left records of ingenious and daring attempts to prevent unwanted pregnancy and childbearing. The range of potions and devices, and the relentness death toll of women desperate to avoid childbirth, bear poignant witness to the age-old longing for reproductive freedom.

Crocodile dung mixed with honey was the principal ingredient of a vaginal suppository (pessary) used by women in ancient Egypt. The Egyptians also fashioned contraceptive tampons from fine wool laced with ground acacia, dates and honey. Papyri have been found with detailed drawings of douching apparatuses and vaginal fumigators to be used before or after sex.

Ancient Chinese women attempted abortion by drinking quicksilver, a powerful poison. In the Middle Ages, European women swallowed lead. Indian women took carrot seeds and the women of northern Canada drank dried beaver testicles in a strong alcoholic solution.

Withdrawal (*coitus interruptus*) dates back at least to the Hebrew Bible, in which Onan, unwilling to obey a command to impregnate his sister-in-law, "spills his seed on the ground." The earliest contraceptive sponge is mentioned in the Talmud, which uses the word "mokh" to describe a spongy substance inserted in the vagina.

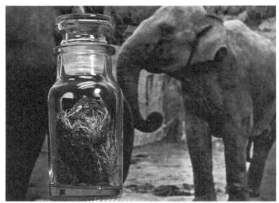

Ortho Pharmaceutical (Canada) Ltd.

Animal dung was a common ingredient in primitive contraceptives. A 9th-century Arabic physician/philosopher, Al-Razi, recommended mixing elephant dung with honey.

The 1st-century A.D. Romans made suppositories from oxgall and serpent fat. Turkish women in the 4th century A.D. used

sponges moistened with diluted lemon juice, while a Mesopotamian recipe of about the same period described a suppository made of pomegranate and gallnut.

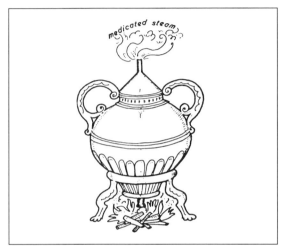

From Finch and Green, *Contraception Through the Ages*, 1963. Courtesy of Charles C. Thomas, Publisher, Springfield, Illinois.

Fumigating the vagina with supposedly contraceptive vapors is a custom that dates back at least to 1850 B.C., when it is mentioned in an Egyptian papyrus. The kettle shown here is from the 16th century.

Ancient Egyptian men used a forerunner of the modern condom, a sheath made of animal membrane. The Chinese fashioned oiled silk paper in a similar manner. In the 18th century in Europe, condoms made of animal intestines served to halt the spread of syphilis as well as to prevent pregnancy. The first rubber condoms were manu-factured about 1880 and latex condoms appeared in the 1930s.

The intrauterine device (IUD) was known to the ancient Arabs, who supposedly put pebbles in camels' uteruses to prevent them from conceiving on long desert

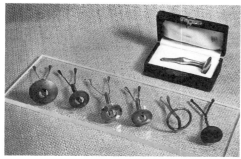

Found in *Abortion in America: The Origins and Evolution of National Policy* by James C. Mohr, Oxford University Press, 1978.

The newspapers of early 19th-century America were filled with advertisements such as this one from the Boston Daily Times *of January 8, 1845. In thinly disguised language, "Madame Drunette" suggests that her French "lunar pills" will induce abortion while her French preventive powders — "for ladies in delicate health" — will prevent pregnancy. Many such potions were highly toxic.*

trips. In the early 1900s, metal IUDs in the shape of wishbones or stems achieved some popularity, but proved

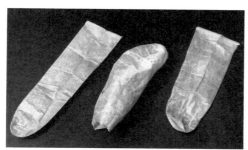

Ortho Pharmaceutical (Canada) Ltd.

A collection of wishbone IUDs from the early 1900s. Behind them, in the case, is a "stem plug," another discontinued form of IUD. These early devices were supposed to be removed, cleaned and reinserted each month. Failure to do this — which was common — led to serious complications and death.

to be quite dangerous and gave IUDs a poor reputation for safety. In the 1930s, the promising Graefenberg ring IUD, an invention of the German doctor Ernst Graefenberg, quickly fell into

disuse as a result of being confused with these earlier, unsafe models.

About 1880, Dr. William Mensinga, a German physician, invented the prototype of the diaphragm that Margaret Sanger discovered on a trip to Europe 35 years later and tried to introduce in the U.S., despite the Comstock laws. Sanger came to prefer a

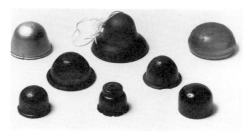

Ortho Pharmaceutical (Canada) Ltd.

The ancient condoms shown here were made of animal membrane or linen, in contrast to the sheer, flexible latex used today.

design created by the Dutch physician, Dr. Aletta Jacobs, which used a spring-fitted rim for easier insertion and removal.

Abortion remedies in use in the American colonies included such poisons as juniper extract, bitter aloes and snakeroot, along with violent exercise such as running and jumping. The newspapers of early 19th-century England and America are replete with advertisements for pills and potions that would supposedly "cure" a woman of an unwanted pregnancy. Primitive and unsanitary surgery was very common;

Sanger wrote of seeing hundreds of mostly immigrant women lined up in lower New York on Saturday nights, risking their lives on kitchen tables for five-dollar abortions.

Similarly, contraceptive sterilization — today a safe and simple procedure that is one of the most popular forms of contraception in the U.S. — evolved from a primitive and violent past. For example, Australian aborigines used a flint knife to split the male urethra partly or completely open, redirecting the course of the semen.

Looking back on the harshness and uncertainties of earlier methods, there can be no doubt that we have come far in the course of this

Ortho Pharmaceutical (Canada) Ltd.

Cervical caps made of rubber, metal and plastic. Designed to fit tightly over the cervix, this method has been in use since the end of the 19th century.

century alone. We owe the relatively safe and effective means of birth control in use today to diligent research and technological advances. But we are also indebted to the determined spirit of those who fought for the tradition of choice and refused to accept any limits on what they could achieve.

Historical Facts and Figures

PLANNED PARENTHOOD FEMALE
CONTRACEPTIVE PATIENTS 1957-1990

Year	New	Continuing	Total
1990	804,057	1,000,666	1,804,723
1989	747,540	975,684	1,723,224
1988	733,001	955,308	1,688,309
1987	729,780	952,576	1,682,356
1986	706,777	906,212	1,612,989
1985	662,120	860,767	1,522,887
1984	637,584	814,183	1,451,767
1983	626,370	759,343	1,385,713
1982	590,480	717,521	1,308,001
1981	575,712	668,228	1,243,940
1980	561,425	641,375	1,202,800
1979	532,542	632,431	1,164,973
1978	542,557	646,090	1,188,647
1977	517,094	613,000	1,130,094
1976	510,098	548,345	1,058,443
1975	520,585	519,323	1,039,908
1974	461,077	458,632	919,709
1973	450,442	402,795	853,237
1972	421,949	317,536	739,485
1971	307,601	248,908	556,509
1970	196,117	211,066	407,183
1969	150,150	195,322	345,472
1968	134,974	188,802	323,776
1967	127,724	182,580	310,304
1966	115,835	164,076	279,911
1965	117,956	158,587	276,543
1964	111,098	124,456	235,554
1963	95,539	123,410	218,949
1962	85,671	96,520	182,191
1961	71,783	88,721	160,504
1960	55,497	67,001	122,498
1959	53,553	63,401	116,954
1958	49,754	60,634	110,388
1957	42,620	58,351	100,971

PLANNED PARENTHOOD FEDERATION OF AMERICA

Chairpersons 1939-Present

Richard N. Pierson, M.D. 1939-1942

J.H.J. Upham, M.D. 1942-1945

The Reverend Cornelius Trowbridge........................... 1945-1948

Charles E. Scribner.. 1948-1950

Eleanor Pillsbury... 1950-1954

Frances Ferguson... 1954-1956

Loraine Campbell.. 1956-1959

Cass Canfield 1959-1962

Donald B. Strauss... 1962-1965

George Lindsay... 1965-1968

Jerome Holland 1968-1969

Joseph Beasley, M.D. 1969-1972

Alan Sweezey, Ph.D. 1972-1975

Henrietta H. Marshall 1975-1978

Frederick C. Smith 1978-1981

Jean Mahoney... 1981-1984

Allan Rosenfield, M.D. 1984-1986

Anne Saunier.. 1986-1989

Kenneth C. Edelin, M.D. 1989-Present

Chief Executives 1939-Present

Margaret Sanger, Honorary President and Chair........... 1939-1962

D. Kenneth Rose, National Director............................. 1939-1948

Dr. Frank Milam, National Director.............................. 1949-1950

William F. Vogt, National Director................................ 1950-1961

Alan F. Guttmacher, M.D., President............................ 1962-1973

    Paul H. Todd, Jr., Chief Executive Officer................ 1966-1969

    John C. Robbins, Chief Executive Officer................ 1969-1973

Jack Hood Vaughn, President....................................... 1974-1975

Henrietta H. Marshall, Acting President........................ 1976-1977

Faye Wattleton, President.. 1978-Present

PLANNED PARENTHOOD FEDERATION OF AMERICA AFFILIATE ANNIVERSARIES

Planned Parenthood of New York City, Inc. 1916

Planned Parenthood of the Rocky Mountains (Aurora, Colorado) 1916

Planned Parenthood League, Inc. (Detroit) 1922

Planned Parenthood Association/Chicago Area (Illinois) 1923

Planned Parenthood of Connecticut, Inc. (New Haven) 1923

Planned Parenthood Center of Syracuse, Inc. (New York) 1925

Planned Parenthood of North East Pennsylvania (Trexlertown) 1926

Planned Parenthood of Houston and Southeast Texas, Inc. 1926

Planned Parenthood Association of Maryland, Inc. (Baltimore) 1927

Planned Parenthood Association of Southeastern Pennsylvania (Philadelphia) 1927

Planned Parenthood League of Massachusetts (Cambridge) 1928

Planned Parenthood/Greater Camden Area (New Jersey) 1928

Planned Parenthood of Greater Cleveland, Inc. (Ohio) 1928

Planned Parenthood Essex County (Newark, New Jersey) 1928

Planned Parenthood of Minnesota (St. Paul) 1928

Planned Parenthood Association of Cincinnati (Ohio) 1929

Planned Parenthood, Alameda/San Francisco (California) 1929

Planned Parenthood of Alabama, Inc. (Birmingham) 1930

Planned Parenthood of Western Pennsylvania (Pittsburgh) 1930

Planned Parenthood of Marin, Sonoma and Mendocino (San Rafael, California) 1930

Planned Parenthood of Rhode Island (Providence) 1931

Planned Parenthood of Delaware (Wilmington) 1931

Planned Parenthood of Mid-Michigan (Ann Arbor) 1932

Planned Parenthood of Central Ohio, Inc. (Columbus) 1932

Planned Parenthood of Lancaster County (Pennsylvania) 1932

Planned Parenthood of Greater Northern New Jersey (Morristown) 1932

Pasadena Planned Parenthood Committee, Inc. (California) 1932

Planned Parenthood of the Capital Region (Harrisburg,Pennsylvania) 1932

Planned Parenthood of Rochester & the Genesee Valley, Inc. (New York) 1932

Planned Parenthood of the St. Louis Region (Missouri) 1932

Planned Parenthood of Buffalo & Erie County, Inc. (New York) 1933

Planned Parenthood of Central Indiana (Indianapolis) 1933

Planned Parenthood of Louisville, Inc. (Kentucky) 1933

Planned Parenthood of Nassau County, Inc. (Hempstead, New York) 1933

Planned Parenthood of Monmouth and Ocean Counties, Inc. (Shrewsbury, New Jersey) 1933

Planned Parenthood of Westchester & Rockland Counties, Inc. (White Plains, New York) 1933

Upper Hudson Planned Parenthood, Inc. (Albany, New York) 1934

Planned Parenthood of Greater Iowa (Des Moines) 1934

Planned Parenthood of Southwestern Indiana, Inc. (Evansville) 1934

Planned Parenthood of Dutchess-Ulster, Inc. (Poughkeepsie, New York) 1934

Planned Parenthood of Southern Arizona, Inc. (Tucson) 1934

Planned Parenthood of Mahoning Valley (Youngstown, Ohio) 1934

Planned Parenthood Committee of Sioux City (Iowa) 1934

Planned Parenthood of Greater Kansas City (Missouri) 1935

Planned Parenthood of Wisconsin (Milwaukee) 1935

Planned Parenthood of West Central Ohio (Springfield) 1935

Planned Parenthood of Omaha-Council Bluffs (Nebraska) 1935

Planned Parenthood Health Services of Northeastern New York (Schenectady) 1935

Planned Parenthood of Seattle-King County (Washington) 1935

Planned Parenthood of Chester County (West Chester, Pennsylvania) 1935

Planned Parenthood of Central Pennsylvania, Inc. (York) 1935

Mountain Maternal Health League Planned Parenthood, Inc. (Berea, Kentucky) 1936

Lexington Planned Parenthood Center, Inc. (Kentucky) 1936

Planned Parenthood of Orange-Sullivan, Inc. (Newburgh, New York) 1936

Passaic County Committee for Planned Parenthood (Paterson, New Jersey) 1936

Planned Parenthood Association of the Mercer Area (Trenton, New Jersey) 1936

Planned Parenthood of Eastern Oklahoma and Western Arkansas, Inc. (Tulsa, Oklahoma) 1936

Planned Parenthood Center of Austin, Inc. (Texas) 1937

Planned Parenthood Center of El Paso, Inc. (Texas) 1937

Planned Parenthood of Niagara County (Niagara Falls, New York) 1937

Planned Parenthood of Central Oklahoma, Inc. (Oklahoma City) 1937

Planned Parenthood of Central and Northern Arizona (Phoenix) 1937

Planned Parenthood of Northwest Ohio, Inc. (Toledo) 1937

Planned Parenthood of Metropolitan Washington, D.C., Inc. 1937

Planned Parenthood of North Texas, Inc. (Fort Worth) 1938

Memphis Planned Parenthood, Inc. (Tennessee) 1938

Planned Parenthood of San Antonio and South Central Texas, Inc. 1939

Planned Parenthood of Central Texas, Inc. (Waco) 1939

Planned Parenthood of Broome and Chenango Counties, Inc. (Binghamton, New York) 1940

Planned Parenthood Association of East Central Illinois (Champaign) 1940

Virginia League for Planned Parenthood, Inc. (Richmond) 1940

Planned Parenthood of the Suffolk County (Commack, New York) 1951

Planned Parenthood Association of Butler County, Inc. (Hamilton, Ohio) 1952

Planned Parenthood of South Texas, Inc. (Corpus Christi) 1958

Planned Parenthood of Central South Carolina, Inc. (Columbia) 1961

Planned Parenthood of East Tennessee, Inc. (Oak Ridge) 1961

Planned Parenthood of Southern New Mexico (Las Cruces) 1962

Planned Parenthood of the Columbia/Willamette (Portland, Oregon) 1962

Planned Parenthood Association of Santa Clara County, Inc. (San Jose, California) 1962

Flint Community Planned Parenthood Association, Inc. (Michigan) 1963

Planned Parenthood Association of Lubbock, Inc. (Texas) 1963

Planned Parenthood Association of Hidalgo County, Inc. (McAllen,Texas) 1963

Planned Parenthood Association of Delaware and Otsego Counties, Inc. (Oneonta, New York) 1963

Planned Parenthood of San Diego and Riverside Counties (California) 1963

Rio Grande Planned Parenthood (Albuquerque, New Mexico) 1964

Planned Parenthood of Southern Indiana, Inc. (Bloomington) 1964

Planned Parenthood of Southeast Iowa (Burlington) 1964

Planned Parenthood Association of Bucks County (Bristol, Pennsylvania) 1964

Planned Parenthood Centers of West Michigan (Grand Rapids) 1964

Tecumseh Area Planned Parenthood Association, Inc. (Lafayette, Indiana) 1964

Planned Parenthood of Northwest/Northeast Indiana, Inc. (Merrillville) 1964

Planned Parenthood Association of Nashville, Inc. (Tennessee) 1964

Planned Parenthood of Sacramento Valley (California) 1964

Planned Parenthood/Orange & San Bernardino Counties, Inc. (Santa Ana, California) 1964

Planned Parenthood of Santa Barbara, Ventura and San Luis Obispo Counties, Inc. (California) 1964

Planned Parenthood Shasta-Diablo (Walnut Creek, California) 1964

Planned Parenthood Association of the Atlanta Area, Inc. (Georgia) 1965

Planned Parenthood of Cameron and Willacy Counties, Inc. (Brownsville, Texas) 1965

Planned Parenthood Association of Miami Valley, Inc. (Dayton, Ohio) 1965

Planned Parenthood of Hawaii (Honolulu) 1965

Planned Parenthood of Northeast Florida, Inc. (Jacksonville) 1965

Planned Parenthood-World Population Los Angeles (California) 1965

Planned Parenthood of North Central Ohio (Mansfield) 1965

Planned Parenthood of East Central Indiana, Inc. (Muncie) 1965

Planned Parenthood of West Texas, Inc. (Odessa) 1965

Planned Parenthood Association of the Greater Peoria Area (Illinois) 1965

Planned Parenthood Association of San Mateo County (California) 1965

Planned Parenthood of Northern New England (Williston, Vermont) 1965

Planned Parenthood of Summit, Portage & Medina Counties (Akron, Ohio) 1966

Planned Parenthood of Stark County (Canton, Ohio) 1966

Planned Parenthood Association of Lane County (Eugene, Oregon) 1966

Planned Parenthood of South Central Michigan (Kalamazoo) 1966

Planned Parenthood of Southwest Florida, Inc. (Sarasota) 1966

Planned Parenthood of North Central Indiana (South Bend) 1966

Planned Parenthood Association of the Mohawk Valley, Inc. (Utica, New York) 1966

Planned Parenthood of Northern New York, Inc. (Watertown) 1966

Planned Parenthood of Central Washington (Yakima) 1966

Planned Parenthood of Alaska (Anchorage) 1966

Planned Parenthood of Decatur, Inc. (Illinois) 1967

Planned Parenthood of the Southern Tier, Inc. (Elmira, New York) 1967

Planned Parenthood of Tompkins County (Ithaca, New York) 1967

Planned Parenthood of Southern Oregon, Inc. (Medford) 1967

Planned Parenthood Association of East Central Ohio (Newark) 1967

Panhandle Planned Parenthood Association, Inc. (Amarillo, Texas) 1968

Planned Parenthood of East Central Georgia, Inc. (Augusta) 1968

Planned Parenthood Association of Southwestern Michigan, Inc. (Benton Harbor) 1969

Intermountain Planned Parenthood, Inc. (Billings, Montana) 1969

Planned Parenthood of Snohomish County (Everett, Washington) 1969

Planned Parenthood of the Finger Lakes, Inc. (Geneva, New York) 1969

Planned Parenthood of Missoula (Montana) 1969

Planned Parenthood of Middlesex County (New Brunswick, New Jersey) 1969

Northern Michigan Planned Parenthood Association (Petoskey) 1969

Mt. Baker Planned Parenthood (Bellingham, Washington) 1970

Planned Parenthood of Southern Piedmont and Carolina Mountains, Inc. (Charlotte, North Carolina) 1970

Planned Parenthood of Central Missouri (Columbia) 1970

Planned Parenthood of Monterey County, Inc. (California) 1970

Planned Parenthood Association of Utah (Salt Lake City) 1970

Planned Parenthood Springfield Area (Ohio) 1970

Planned Parenthood of San Joaquin Valley, Inc. (Stockton, California) 1970

Planned Parenthood of Walla Walla (Washington) 1970

Planned Parenthood of Southeast Ohio (Athens) 1971

Planned Parenthood Association of Idaho, Inc. (Boise) 1971

Planned Parenthood of Central California (Fresno) 1971

Marquette-Alger Planned Parenthood, Inc. (Michigan) 1971

Northern Adirondack Planned Parenthood, Inc. (Plattsburgh, New York) 1971

Planned Parenthood of Northern Nevada, Inc. (Reno) 1971

Planned Parenthood of Santa Cruz County (California) 1971

Planned Parenthood of Spokane & Whitman Counties (Washington) 1971

Planned Parenthood of Kansas (Wichita) 1971

Planned Parenthood of Southern Nevada, Inc. (Las Vegas) 1972

Planned Parenthood of Pierce County (Tacoma, Washington) 1972

Planned Parenthood of the Palm Beach Area, Inc. (West Palm Beach, Florida) 1972

Planned Parenthood of Lincoln (Nebraska) 1973

Planned Parenthood North Central Florida, Inc. (Gainesville) 1974

Planned Parenthood of Northeast Missouri, Inc. (Kirksville) 1974

Planned Parenthood of the Central Ozarks (Rolla, Missouri) 1974

Planned Parenthood Association of Greater Miami, Inc. 1975

Six Rivers Planned Parenthood (Eureka, California) 1975

Planned Parenthood of Southeastern Virginia, Inc. (Hampton) 1976

Planned Parenthood of the Blue Ridge, Inc. (Roanoke, Virginia) 1976

Planned Parenthood of Central Florida, Inc. (Lakeland) 1979

Planned Parenthood of South Palm Beach & Broward Counties, Inc. (Florida) 1980

Planned Parenthood of Linn County, Inc. (Cedar Rapids, Iowa) 1980

Planned Parenthood of the Capitol and Coast, Inc. (Raleigh, North Carolina) 1981

Planned Parenthood of the Triad, Inc. (Winston-Salem, North Carolina) 1981

Planned Parenthood of Orange and Durham Counties, Inc. (Chapel Hill, North Carolina) 1982

Planned Parenthood of Dallas & Northeast Texas, Inc. 1982

Planned Parenthood of Tallahassee, Inc. (Florida) 1983

Planned Parenthood of Louisiana (New Orleans) 1983

Planned Parenthood of Greater Arkansas (Little Rock) 1986

Planned Parenthood of the Low Country, Inc. (Hilton Head Island, South Carolina) 1989

Please note: Establishment dates of affiliates are based on information provided by affiliates.

SOURCES

Primary Sources

Interviews conducted in 1990-91 with: Dr. Joan Babbott, Winfield Best, Kenneth C. Edelin, M.D., Heather Estes, Ellen Fairchild, Douglas Gould, Naomi Gray, Lee Minto, Miriam Manisoff, Alfred F. Moran, Eve Paul, Harriet F. Pilpel, Fannie Porter, Larry Rodick, Jeannie I. Rosoff, Dr. Irving Rust, Mark Salo, Kay Scott, Pamela Veerhusen, Faye Wattleton, Thomas Webber, Eloise Whitten

Planned Parenthood Sources

Family Planning International Assistance Annual Report, 1989.

INsider, PPFA Newsletter, 1987-1991.

Nattier, Linda White, *Planned Parenthood of St. Louis: The First 50 Years,* November 1982.

Planned Parenthood Association of Miami Valley, "Ohio [Dayton]: Planned Parenthood Association of Miami Valley," one-page unpublished history, 1979.

Planned Parenthood Federation of America Annual Reports, 1954-1990.

PPFA Fact Sheets, 1989-1990.

PPFA Interregional Statistical Report, 1969.

PPFA Service Reports, 1987-1990.

Planned Parenthood League of Connecticut, "Planned Parenthood 1923-1983."

Planned Parenthood League of Massachusetts, *PPLM Reports,* Spring 1974, Number 24.

Planned Parenthood News, 1952-69.

Planned Parenthood *News Exchange,* March 1944-May/June 1952.

Planned Parenthood *News Letter,* April-May 1942.

Planned Parenthood of Alabama, Inc., "History of Planned Parenthood of Alabama, Inc." two-page unpublished history, October 1990.

Planned Parenthood of Maryland, "PPM's First 60 Years," Spring 1987.

Planned Parenthood of New York City, "Making History Happen: The First 20 Years of Planned Parenthood of New York City," 1986.

Planned Parenthood of Seattle-King County, "50 Years of Progress...And a Long Way to Go," 1985.

Planned Parenthood of the Atlanta Area, "Window of Opportunity: 25th Anniversary Publication," October 1989.

Planned Parenthood of the Rocky Mountains, "Colorado [Denver]: Rocky Mountain Planned Parenthood," two-page unpublished history, 1979.

Planned Parenthood Review, 1981-86.

Rein, Martin, "An Organizational Analysis of a National Agency's Local Affiliates in their Community Contexts," 1961.

Other Secondary Sources

Finch, B.E. and Hugh Green, *Contraception Through the Ages* (Springfield, Illinois: Charles C. Thomas) 1963.

Jaffe, Frederick S., "Family Planning, Public Policy and Intervention Strategy," *Journal of Social Issues,* October 1967.

Kennedy, David M., *Birth Control in America: The Career of Margaret Sanger* (New Haven, Connecticut: Yale University Press) 1970.

Mohr, James, *Abortion in America: The Origins and Evolution of National Policy 1800-1900* (New York: Oxford University Press) 1978.

Reed, James, *The Birth Control Movement and American Society: From Private Vice to Public Virtue* (Princeton, New Jersey: Princeton University Press) 1984.

Rock, John, *The Time Has Come: A Catholic Doctor's Proposal to End the Battle Over Birth Control* (New York: Knopf) 1963.

Rosoff, Jeannie I., "The Politics of Birth Control," *Family Planning Perspectives,* Nov.-Dec. 1988, 20, 6, 312-320.

Sanger, Margaret, *An Autobiography* (New York: W.W. Norton) 1938.

Skuy, Percy, "A History of Contraception: How Far Have We Really Come?" *Canadian Pharmaceutical Journal,* Nov. 1976, *109,* 11.

Valenza, Charles, "Was Margaret Sanger a Racist?" *Family Planning Perspectives,* Jan.-Feb. 1985, 17, 1, 44-46.

Many thanks to the treasure-keepers: Gloria Roberts and Harriet Schick at the Katharine Dexter McCormick Memorial Library of Planned Parenthood Federation of America; Jeanne Swinton, former librarian at the Abraham Stone Memorial Library of Planned Parenthood of New York City; and Margery Sly and Susan Boone at the Sophia Smith Collection of Smith College.

Writer: Jane Alpert

Editor: Barbara Snow

Designer: Dale Tangeman

Photo Researcher: Helena Clarke